Permission

WHAT OTHERS ARE SAYING ABOUT *PERMISSION*

If you have ever felt stuck between the societal archetypes of the good girl and switched on woman...

If you've ever wondered if wanting 'vanilla' sex makes you boring...

If the need for your experience as a sexual woman to be validated...

Read Permission.

In Permission, Lauren offers guidance and practical wisdom that will help you to explore your relationship with sex, intimacy and your personal health. It will cultivate, support and liberate your feminine reclamation so that you will never seek, or most importantly, *need* permission for your own sexual expression ever again.

—Lisa Lister
Bestselling author of *Witch*,
Love Your Lady Landscape and *Code Red*

Lauren White's breakthrough first book, Permission, is an affirming, wise and illuminating read which unpacks the many reasons why women seek external validation, rather than looking internally and trusting in their own permission giving abilities. Through research, anecdote and deep personal revelation White explores the complex relationships women have with their own bodies and sexualities, arguing that true liberation comes from permission giving within.

—Nina Funnell
Walkley award winning journalist and author

Permission is a big sigh of relief. Lauren White upends many of the progressive sex scripts and tips we've grown accustomed to and invites women, instead, to be who they are as they are. Out with the pressure. Welcome to your own path to being switched on.

—Molly Caro May
Author of *Body Full of Stars: Female Rage*
and My Passage Into Motherhood

I read this book at just the right time, seriously the timing was spooky. Too many of us fill our lives with empty pleasures or things, instead of embracing our inner sexuality. Lauren's book helped me realised I can acknowledge my inner good girl and still be a sexy little minx all at the same time. Liberating, sensitive and incredibly thought provoking. Read it now.

—Kate Toon

SEO lover, award winning copywriter, author and speaker

"Permission is fundamental to liberation. You're free when you live as you choose.... You're free when you live your life from a place of wholehearted giving to yourself and giving to others without the constant self sacrifice, martyr mode and burnout.' Having recently thrown off a life of constant self sacrifice, being in martyr mode and burning myself out (right through to multiple organ failure), I can attest to Lauren's assertion that you're only truly free when you give yourself permission to live as you choose. Giving up the 9-5, societal expectations and familial norms that have existed for generations is what I finally allowed me to create and enjoy a fully liberated life - I can't recommend it highly enough!

—Maria Doyle

Teacher Trainer and Curriculum Developer

"*Permission* made me stop. It's not often that a book creates a life changing experience for you, *Permission* did this for me. Throughout the chapters I felt myself stop and look inwards on who I am, what I really want and who I am. I have always been the good girl, the well-behaved person that had it together. I fitted the mould that was expected of me and from this I feel that I lost a part of me and my voice. Reading *Permission* has allowed me to create a space to reflect in awards and see what I need for all areas of my life."

—Lauren June

Business Development Strategist

Permission

PERSONAL LIBERATION FOR SWITCHED ON WOMEN

LAUREN WHITE

Permission: Personal Liberation for Switched On Women

All names and identifying details of the individuals in this book have been changed to protect their privacy.

Cover photo and author photo by Nicole Barralet
Cover design by Anna Dower
Book design by Maureen Cutajar

To Yvette and Sylvia.
Created perfectly by sex and heart.

ACKNOWLEDGEMENTS

Thank you to the blank page for holding the word *PERMISSION* in early 2017 and just letting it sit there to marinate for a little while longer. This was one of the most beautiful lessons in timing, surrender and trust. I'm no longer 'trying to trust'.

To Ed for being the most supreme permission wingman I could ever ask for. I hold no regrets about my verbal prayer to the big wide world to marry you one day. You continue to teach me so much about what I desire (and resist) most – the ultimate permission granter in love and life through your two favourite words: *why not?*

To Lisa Lister for giving the most succinct and timely suggestions and writing prompts so that this high achiever was juiced up but never overwhelmed. For being one of the few editors on earth that can recommend self-pleasure as a companion to writing and one of the very, very few that would work by honouring both our internal cycles and those of mama earth. Collaborating with you also instilled a little more of the quiet middle finger in me – constantly edging me closer to my own sovereignty. This creative experience was so empowering and liberating – you are one of my dearest permission granters and I love you fiercely.

To Sylvia Plath for hearing my multiple calls and allowing me to source the words as I needed them. We both write alone and with fervour.

To the women I love and know personally in family, life and biz – Mum, Sah, Pen, Heather, Suzy, Tina, Kateoy, Sim, Kirsty, Fran, George, Neens, Anna Dower, Yvonne Lumsden, Nicole Barralet, Alyssa Martin and all my friends that weave in and out so organically.

To Hugs Café for the steady stream of long blacks and generosity in space to write (and actual hugs).

To Nicole Mathieson for creating the anchor for the *Permission to have trauma* chapter through your heartfelt idea and generous contribution. I believe this gave *Permission* a much needed spine to support her.

To every client I have ever had the privilege of listening to. Thank you for sharing your stories with me. I'm still listening.

To the women that I am yet to meet that keep moving as permission granters despite adversity, disadvantage, oppression, homophobia, transphobia, misogyny, trauma and pain… whether behind closed doors for one or standing in front of millions…you are creating a ripple of change.

CONTENTS

PART 1

PROLOGUE

MY WHOLE LIFE I CRAVED PERMISSION.

My problem wasn't that I needed others to tell me what to do.

That's direction.

That's guidance.

That's advice.

What *I* needed was confirmation that I should go for what I want.

For far too long, I questioned others as to what my next move was going to be when it was glaringly obvious that I already knew the answer to my own problem.

This tendency of mine was all too often heralded as an inability to make decisions.

I'm telling you right now, that making decisions was *never* the problem. That was the cover story.

I always knew the answer. I just wanted everyone else's approval first.

From doctors to teachers to mentors to co-workers, friends, books and lovers, I have looked ever-outward to get the green light to do, and be, exactly who I was born to be. That dependent approach worked for a long time.

Until it didn't.

My forays into the world of human sexuality highlighted to me that looking outward was *not* going to get me closer to owning my sexuality. I couldn't be both seeking permission *and* be empowered. There's always a payoff.

In fact, it all came down to this: **how can I truly be who I am if I always need someone else to say *permission granted*?**

Strangely, waiting with baited breath to hear permission being granted was rarely about the big compelling life decisions like, what career path I should take, or where I should live. The anxiety of approval worked backwards in me, and it was the small decisions that caused me the most angst and required a much more thorough de-brief. And if I couldn't consult someone at the time, then I would seek permission *after* the event.

That's when I knew my need for permission ran deep.

When I was faced with a choice and I responded by making my decision, yet I *still* wanted, and needed, confirmation from someone that it was the right decision to make.

Maybe handling the big decisions of life without a permission granter was easier because the pool of possible decisions was narrower. Flip it around to the smaller stuff though, and the need for permission ruthlessly infiltrated all the irrelevant parts that seemed so desperately important to me at the time.

Cast your imagination into the quintessential restaurant scene, and I was the woman sitting there *umming* and *ahhhing* over what to order. This tendency of mine to deliberate over what I ordered in restaurants got so painful for my family to endure that there would be serious tension when it was my turn to say what I wanted. All of those repetitive occasions culminated in one big fight between my Dad and I. There I was, at 17, so far enjoying our father-daughter Bali trip where my inability to decide what I would order for dinner was so deliberated that he cracked it. Words were exchanged about how I can never make a decision and I had little to throw back to that one. I sobbed at the table; snot dripping down all the way through some forgettable noodle dish. In the midst of being stonewalled by him, it felt fitting to rebelliously spend the rest of the evening all angsty with my journal and an overpriced bottle of Jacobs Creek Chardonnay.

Let's look a little closer at that one. It may not look like it but I always knew what I wanted on the menu that night, just *what would other people (in this case my Dad) think of what I wanted? What was going to be the answer that pleased them?*

This is all pesky, right? Small. Insignificant. Yet, it's the small and insignificant that is so telling of what condition the more personal facets of our identity are in. I've found that, if we struggle with the seemingly small things, it'll usually cascade through to our most intimate encounters.

You may have already guessed what I'm about to say next.

Amidst all the little permission granting I required, the part of me that needed the most permission, and I'm talking by far, by a long shot and in a slow burn sort of way, was my libido.

It needed this because it's been up against some pretty serious stop signs, causing me to taste the flavours of *falling short* and *not enough* many times over. No wonder it was confused and misdirected, it wasn't being given the permission that it needed to move towards what feels good.

Maturity, marriage, mamahood and working with women taught me that the best things in life are a slow burn and obtaining the permission to run with my very high libido for life was no different. If I allowed it, time would permit its evolution.

Since immersing myself in the, equally enlightening, equally befuddling, learning that only human sexuality can provide, I am now held in a cocoon where I only seek permission when I'm truly stuck and I can't see out of my own scope. In the inevitability of human dilemma, and as a helper that needs help sometimes, I'm going to need to seek permission from other people. Yet rather than this being a case of need and dependency like it used to be, the flavour is now occasional-requirement.

Sometimes I wonder, maybe, just maybe, if we weren't raised to be 'good girls', then external permission wouldn't hold such appeal.

And us good girls love permission because it reduces the risk that we'll get something wrong or make a mistake. I've done this when I valued a superior's expertise over my own internal compass and I'm now left questioning whether those 'certain outcomes' were worth more than the liberation of working it out for myself.

I want you to know, straight up, that when you start giving yourself permission, you don't automatically lose touch with your good girl.

My good girl is a humbling asset that I need to draw upon to get shit done because she values loyalty, following through with what she said she would do, and completing tasks to the best of her ability. All of this is magnified when her actions are going to have an impact, or follow on effect, to others – there's no way she can handle the possibility of being seen as someone who doesn't finish what they said they would. That fear of being perceived as lazy or unhelpful drives her over the finish line every time.

I love my inner good girl and all that she has done for me. It's just that I reached a point where I didn't want her need for external permission to dominate my life anymore.

That's what *Permission* is all about: keeping the desirable aspects of your good girl, your need to control, and your tendency to be serious and choosy, whilst still allowing your libido to have its fullest expression.

What brought you to needing to become your own permission granter might not have been something glaringly obvious on the surface, it might have been:

- This general discomfort about sex that you can't quite pinpoint
- A feeling that you are holding back in sex but you don't know why
- Having trouble expressing what you like and need in the bedroom
- An inkling that more intimacy and vulnerability is possible
- Realising that you are often looking to others to validate you
- A feeling like sex is something you should do rather than something you want to do
- Not getting what your body is capable of or feeling like it is faulty
- A nudge that saying yes to doing lots of things (or all the things) in life is sapping your sexual energy

All of that might not seem possible to understand and move through, but I'm living proof that it is.

Let me show you…

Lauren xo

INTRODUCTION

CAN I ASK YOU SOMETHING?

Do you seek permission?

Not just to be polite, or to adhere to niceties, but to validate nearly every move or decision you make?

I'm talking about seeking permission when you are...

Needing something commonplace or ordinary in the office?

Glancing over the menu in the restaurant?

Trying to solve your problems with your friends?

Making a small financial decision?

Filling in your parents on your life plans?

Getting warm in the bedroom?

Constantly using words like, *can I, may I, would it be alright if, should I, do you think, excuse me, do you mind if I*... as the start of what you say again and again (and again and again?)

I want you to know there is nothing wrong with you needing permission.

You are not defective, broken, useless, stupid, or whatever other harsh word you might address yourself with, when you lose your way and need guidance.

You are enough as you are right now (and that includes your sexuality).

So if you're asking yourself where your libido/sex drive/sexuality or mojo is, it's possible that you've become focused on what you lack, or you think you don't have, so naturally, you ask others to fill in the gaps. Doing that keeps the attention on what you aren't enough of and how you need *more.*

Only that, your problem isn't that you aren't sexual enough, it's just that you haven't given yourself permission to access your sexual power. Yet.

I can relate. My inner sexual world and expression is likely not too different to yours. We probably started off hearing similar crappy and shameful messages about female sexuality. The only difference is that I've learnt to drown out the white noise and increase the volume on all the stuff in life that feels good and that's what being your own permission granter is all about.

I was someone who had my shit together in all the areas of my life but didn't dare ask for what I wanted in the bedroom. I always felt my sexuality wasn't enough, and needed to be more, so I avoided being vulnerable in sex because I honestly thought it made me look weak and fragile. Instead of risking that, I defaulted to following the leader, which was always the other person.

I wasn't born a Tantric goddess and I haven't experienced a straight, ascending, line of libido improvement as time goes on, because life doesn't usually play well with straight lines. Before I started learning about sex, my connection to it was patchy at best. It was on…it was off (a lot more than it was on) and what this looked like was sexual energy that spilt out into all the wrong places (and people) and a whole lot of confusion.

I didn't understand that in suppressing this fire in me for so long and living life as *a good girl, a smart good and a good wife,* so faithfully that I would be sitting there at age 27 very… confused. On the outside, the boxes of my life had been ticked, I loved my husband Ed, but internally, I felt so shutdown and closed off.

I wanted it but I didn't want it. I hated being vulnerable and loathed being seen this way in the bedroom. I judged all of sex as, kind of, negative unless I had a few drinks and suddenly had the permission to let loose. Sound familiar?

At the heart of it all, I didn't have a fulfilling sex life and it didn't create flow between us as a couple. I kept defaulting to having Ed work it all out for me and being plain passive about my own role in our sex life.

Learning about my sexuality formally, and informally, changed all that. Eventually.

I slowly matured, owned my role in my marriage, and got into the very raw business of unearthing my libido *for me.* These days, I still have lapses into an un-libidinous life at times like when stress is high, or during pregnancy and postpartum recovery, but these lapses don't last for long and I know how to come back to my libido quickly. Not that it's about speed, more about clarity and efficiency with a lot less anxiety.

It's an honour to say the words to you that I WISH someone had said to me:

You don't need an external permission slip for anything anymore.

Permission already exists inside of you. You don't need to live with sexual repression, boredom and frustration. It's definitely not too late to change. As long as you show up, and ask yourself the necessary questions, permission will edge you out of awkwardness and inhibition. More importantly, you don't need to wait for an external source to tell you when the time is right and what the next move will be. Self-sourcing permission isn't reliant on an external source – it's solely reliant on you.

One of the key traits of switched-on women is that we are impatient. So, if you are feeling that way, can I ask that you use your impatience for good, and become your own permission granter right now?

When I devotedly followed my own internal green light I never looked back.

Sometimes I paused, and stepped to the side for a while, but I never went back.

My deepest hope is that the same will ring true for you.

How self-sourcing permission shows up

I like that permission doesn't always happen in the traditional way of us going to someone and asking a question in order to get an authoritative answer. Sometimes it likes to surprise us, like when we are in the audience listening to a speaker, chatting with a friend on our couch, or with a colleague in the office kitchen, and suddenly permission just inserts itself into the conversation. One moment you are nodding your head on autopilot and the next minute you are having a deep revelation.

This is one of the key reasons why we need to keep in constant conversation with other women. Our stories have so much power to grant permission.

It will happen to me a handful of times every year. There I am, listening to or reading another woman's story and it begins gently unfurling something within me that I have been holding on to with serious tenacity. A notion. A concept. A 'truth'. And then she says the opposite. A huge opening appears. Sometimes, I audibly gasp with a sharp inhalation.

Fuck. How did I not come to that conclusion on my own?

Bam! Why didn't I flip that script around?

Being immersed in women's work means that I'll always need to keep witnessing and learning from other women as there is no end point to our sacred contract to stick together. Personally, as long as I continue to learn from other women in all sorts of situations and contexts, I will live more of my life as my own self-sourcing permission granter. I assure you, it all gets easier and becomes more natural if you keep going and you always nurture your connections with other women. Always.

There is this magical moment when you give yourself permission and you know that it is self-sourcing. Fuck it feels powerful.

You'll know when you are giving yourself permission because it feels full and ripe as it reverberates around your body. Impenetrable. You trust the next move you are about to make (or not make) with every fibre of your being because you trust you.

The biggest indicator that you're ready to give yourself permission is when you are asking questions that you already know the answer to. Also, seeking answers from multiple sources, and concocting silent rebuttals in your mind, is a flashing light that you don't need external permission.

Because you already know.

Moving permission from being externally sourced to internally sourced

I believe self-sourced permission makes us bold and that being bold means running the risk of fucking up. This is a gamble that I didn't even have to consider when I had someone else telling me what the next move was, but then I started to see the other persons answer as a bigger gamble, like a 'results may vary' kind of gamble, whereas my own permission granting started to feel like the more certain of the two.

Not that being bold has resulted in life being completely smooth. The moments where I've moved full steam ahead with my own permission, without checking if maybe it's the right thing to do, mean that I've made a mistake or two (or three or four). In the name of giving myself permission I have made changes to my life, relationships, and business, that have usually had the air of 'fuck it…I trust it will all come back to me'.

Unsurprisingly, it hasn't always worked, but I have gotten much closer to my joy this way than by gritting my teeth and scrambling to reach my own sky-high standards. Turns out that those standards are usually dependent on external validation that takes me full circle back to needing another's permission.

Liberation can't be dependent on what everyone else thinks.

The reality is that permission has been an ongoing process of giving myself this gift over and over. I still occasionally fall into the trap of waiting for someone else to give me the green light, usually another woman, because I value the personal reflection that she can provide. I stayed in this gear for years until the words "I was waiting for you to give me permission" stumbled from my mouth and across the virtual room to my business mentor Anna.

It was two months before I started writing *Permission* and that moment felt equally heavy with despair and promise. I had to actually say that in order to feel the cost that external permission seeking was having on me. Even as the words "I was waiting for you to give me permission" arose, I distinctly recall thinking to myself – *I really want her to give me this specific answer right now.* My desire was concrete and this short cut in asking her wasn't actually saving me (or her) any time. And that was the last time I sought permission from her, from anyone really. I felt the sadness of seeking the answers outside of my, very tired, body and finally acknowledged that the moment that I feel tempted to ask the question of 'what should I do?' I instead need to ask myself, 'what answer do I want to hear?'

I started to analyse this a little more closely by breaking down the historical chain of events. A problem occurs and I immediately think, *I don't know the answer.* I grab my phone to go and ask someone I see as being wiser than me. I'm reactionary because the stress of the problem, regardless of size, consumes all my attention and presence. Problems used to take me into hyper-arousal, which feeds my hyper-arousal, which never allowed me to ask myself a question because I was on high alert and struggled to concentrate. I started to notice that doing this on repeat was having certain people tire of my questions and, I knew deep in my bones, that I was pushing the boundaries of their good graces. In the beginning, they were helping me, later on I was just cutting a corner so that I could quickly move through overwhelm.

Until I felt how irritating my default to seeking external permission was, I struggled to curb this habit. Looking at every woman I respected, what I really wanted to be was radiant and magnetic but in reality I was pestering and being irritating. That ravine felt huge and it irked me. Neediness felt like an old pattern in the form of a young girl. In order to get to magnetic and radiant, I had to give neediness the flick and stand up a little for myself by myself.

I quickly weaned myself off going straight to others for answers. I had a choice to stay put in neediness or to move on gracefully into sovereignty.

The allure of being magnetic meant sovereignty won.

Now, as soon as I have a problem, I slow myself down and I ask if I need genuine help or if I'm being needy. I decide I don't have to be reactionary like I used to be. I go inward first and ask myself – *what answer do I want to hear?* Doing this consistently, for over a year, has given me laser-focused insight into what I truly want and allows me to become self-sourcing. If I'm still stuck after asking myself this, then I know it's safe for me to ask for help and that I can surrender to support. Since I learnt to slow down a little, and be less reactionary, I can distinctly feel the occasions where I'm out of my depth and know that new learnings will come from another woman's wisdom. Her wisdom will show me what I'm struggling to grasp.

I hope you're beginning to see that eradicating permission from other people entirely isn't the end goal here. Perhaps, right now in your life, are you seeking permission when you *feel* you are out of your depth? Is it possible to look back and observe the difference between the times where you actually needed permission and the times where you purely lacked confidence? I believe that when you feel these differences for yourself first, you can then start to reduce your need in seeking an external permission granter. When you know what your actual needs are, the permission cycle can then break to become self-sourcing rather than externally dependent.

Permission is not always a signal to go

As you progress through this book, keep in mind that permission isn't always about needing a green light to go, or to get closer to something. The amber light to slow down and the red light to stop are equally as important. If there's a high achiever, or good girl, inside of you, she might like things to move fast and to hit goals quickly with little or no rest in-between. In this case, the permission you need might not be a green light to go, it will be an amber light to slow down or a red light to stop. In whatever way permission presents itself to you, it needs to be your own gateway to liberation and personal health. You'll know it's the right medicine for you in that moment because you will feel its relief when you meet it.

There are a million external green lights so choose which ones match the frequency of your own internal green light.

Even though permission is a simple construct that we can conceptualise as green, amber, and red, sometimes it goes a little bit beyond this. What I mean is that sometimes permission needs its own permission.

Gaining permission, or having it granted, does not mean that you have to follow through with an action. You are free to leave the offers, suggestions, and all the well-meaning advice and walk away from it in your own direction. This moves in the form of: *I give myself permission to not use another's, or my own, permission.* Take a moment. Breathe THAT in.

The words of permission

Permission is a sensitive creature. I've seen it work more effectively when it's invited by words that are thoughtful, invoking, yet strangely powerful. Through my ever-growing love of language, and working with women at their most vulnerable, I've learnt that an entire message can be missed because of the deterring nature of one word. Other times a message can suddenly penetrate a tough exterior because of the possibility of one word.

Throughout *Permission*, I have attempted to use the most inclusive words that I can – words that invite you in rather than shut you out. The space that permission calls for us to inhabit requires words that are both clear and soft.

In the theme of this, I have chosen to use the following words and concepts for the vast majority of the book:

Libido instead of *sexuality*
Enjoyment instead of *pleasure*
Curious instead of *desire*
Releasing instead of *letting go*
Self-centred instead of *selfish*

I use these words to consistently draw us back to creating an earthy, rock solid, foundation of *yes* rather than floating high into a kind of false transcendence. Words that feel too far away from where you are can cause you to check-out. In all sincerity, I'd rather you be here, be grounded, and not floating away and feeling lost.

How to use this book

I have a sneaking suspicion that you are smart and switched on. Those modes are probably pretty easy for you. I'm saying that as a gesture of trust for what lies ahead. I trust that you will have your own way of absorbing and interpreting these upcoming nuggets of permission because that is the whole point. True permission is about being discerning and taking what you need, when you need it, rather than blindly swallowing the prescription. There's nothing in here that you have to believe or follow. When you integrate permission at your own discretion, you are transforming primal wisdom into something intensely personal.

And nothing is more personal than sex.

At its core, permission is simple. It asks that you cut through all the noise, flashing lights and big concepts that are out there in life, and especially in the personal growth world, so that you can nuzzle down into that sweet spot where intimate knowledge meets your individuality. You might have already noticed that tabloid sex advice completely misses this need for women and that's why it rarely moves or liberates you.

Are you with me when I say we will be ditching vapid for real right now?

Because permission wants you to be real and it wants to provide you with unwavering support. Not only will it always be there for you but, if you forget about it and need to fall back, it will be your safety net that magically appears.

You can drop out of touch with self-sourcing permission and come back. You can always come back.

And if you do drop out, or check out, and anxiety begins to arise in your body, I invite you to place your feet on solid ground, or on your bed, and say to yourself, *I'm safe. I'm safe.*

I've got me. I trust me. There's a lot more on safety and trust to come. Self-sourcing permission depends on it.

In the true spirit of permission, I gave myself permission to not include a plethora of formal exercises, practices or journal prompts within the pages of this book. I've done this because I hope you are moved by the power of simplicity – that absorbing the words you are about to read is...enough.

I trust that you'll learn just by being here and that you'll begin to ask and answer your own questions.

Yes, you will learn but you are also going to stall

Throughout your metamorphosis from external permission seeker to internal permission granter, you will ebb and flow, drop and rebound. When you notice yourself growing and then stalling, one thing you can ask yourself is, 'what can I learn right now?' Permission is the perfect incubator to learn in and chances are you will:

- Resist
- Sabotage
- Stop (what I will reframe as a *pause*)
- Check-out
- Fuck up and
- Be triggered

You'll do these things because you're human and beautifully flawed. You'll do these things because you can't put your curated resume of life next to your sex life as it stands right now. They are incomparable and there is no linear trajectory or check boxes in your sex life (much to this high-achievers dismay).

Permission may gently tinker with your ego and your defences. If fear has held the reins on your libido and sex life so far, you will already be very familiar, maybe even friendly, with your defences. They have protected you for so long and for compelling reasons. Considering cutting the cord with your defences is daunting, but there's a chance, if you're reading this book, that you've reached a stalemate with them and you're looking for the next stellar move.

Your inhibitions need to drop gently so that you can open up.

Permission is less *what you should do in the bedroom* and more *this is what will give you the best opportunity to actually get into the bedroom*. When your internal guard is up, declaring *no* and permission to be sexual is absent from your life, all the sex tips and advice in the world will fall pretty flat. That's because our ability to take in information is reduced when we're in a state of fear.

You have to feel safe and aligned with being sexual in order to become sexual.

The sense of safety has to come first. The feeling of it being possible to be sexual can come second. Without these, you'll very possibly be pushing, striving and forcing desire and arousal. Tellingly, most women know how that tryst in the bedroom plays out – you're in your head and your body is devoid of pleasure. Instead of being present, you are absent.

> *It's time to unravel all of the conditioning, rules and dogma that have governed your sex life for too long.*

> *It's time to have your head, heart and body be in a symbiotic relationship, not acting like opposing forces.*

> *It's time for you to declare your worthiness of being a sexual woman in a way that is true for you.*

Know that I'm not here to change you

Most importantly, wherever you're at in your permission granting journey, please know that I'm not here to change you. I believe that your libido is already an all-knowing unique entity that simply needs the lid taken off so it can breathe and move. True permission moves like an undercurrent to gently crack open what is already inside of you. All that vibrancy is there, for all of us, it's really just a matter of whether we are willing to allow ourselves to be radiant or, more personally, whether we feel we are worthy of being radiant.

Lastly, try not to get caught up on how many occasions in your life you have sought any kind of external permission up until this point. Resist the urge to spiral into 'I should have known better' territory before you even let yourself become your own permission granter. Know that you are a power source, that you have done your best, and that thinking that other people, or systems, always knew what was best for you first was simply a habit at play.

As your confidence in self-sourcing permission increases, the need to look outward to others in a way that is needy or dependent will reduce considerably. It's pure math (well, more like *feeling* math).

It's time to open and get liberated.

Permission granted.

ONE

Becoming your own Permission Granter

I'LL 'FESS UP. In my formative years, being my own permission granter didn't hold that much appeal.

Receiving permission from outside of myself was easy because the parameters and expectations were already established. In the safety of every institution I studied and worked in, all I ever had to do was sit back and digest the pre-packaged permission that asked for nothing more on my end of things. I relished sticking to the rules and the rewards that came from being a good girl who was trustworthy and always showed up to do "the right thing". Doing life that way was comfortable and gave me a sense of certainty but, over time, that comfort got kind of stale and I was instinctively craving the certain satisfaction that could only come from doing things the *Lauren* way. The more wisdom I absorbed about sex, the more I understood that less individuality and effort usually meant less satisfaction, and less satisfaction meant that I became idle and restless.

When I'm idle and restless, I'm not tapping into my power.

All of this makes me think of the 1950's housewife prototype that had all the guesswork of her life taken from her. She was told what her place was and how she was to act within her prescribed role. All decision-making and permission granting was externally thrust upon her. With the light of her power dimmed, she had this excess fire that she didn't know how to channel. All of the usual activities and pastimes of her era just didn't satiate her. So…

She wondered if she needed to try harder.

She wondered if there's something wrong with her.

She wondered why everything she ever wanted had her nervous system dialled up to high voltage.

Since the 1950's, women have encountered a new dilemma.

There's a kind of ambiguity and murkiness that comes with all that's now possible for a woman to source from within herself. Deep down, we know we can be our own permission granters but we stall by wondering where we need to start, what we need to do, and how it's all going to look. Deep, deep, down we question: *what will people think?* Cue slumping to the floor declaring: *it's all too fucking hard. Will someone just tell me what to do?*

In moments like these, you're going to need a little boost to step into becoming your own permission granter because, in the thick of all the personal growth mess, you might forget that there is absolute gold awaiting you. Now, this gold isn't just a nice-to-have, it's the element that women thirst for when they sit down before me wanting to have a better sex life, only they don't yet know that this is what will truly satisfy them.

Your permission granting journey will need a solid foundation – a purpose and reminder in the times that it loses its appeal. The following is what I call the golden trifecta of permission granting.

THE GOLDEN TRIFECTA OF PERMISSION GRANTING

PERMISSION GRANTING
Informs, creates and influences

OWNERSHIP
+
ALIGNMENT
+
SOVEREIGNTY
↓
LIBERATION
=
PERSONAL HEALTH

#1 OWNERSHIP

Permission is a major exercise in raising awareness. It's the first step, to stirring everything up, to edging closer to your liberation, but it needs allies to move it from simply knowing or understanding to full activation.

In my own life, the biggest propeller of permission is ownership. After that initial stirring that permission provides me with, I need constant motion to elevate me into becoming what it is that I want to be and feel. Permission can come to me when I'm stuck and in stasis but actually shifting my habits and being something different is where ownership has the chance to shine.

Internal permission relies on repetition for reinforcement and that's why it needs to happen again and again and again from within.

Yet when you move into a state of ownership, you do it once and you never forget.

You front up in the world exactly as you want to because you own it.

Have you ever heard someone say: "*she owned it*"?

When I see a woman living life exactly how she is destined to, in all of her unique ways, I think *she owns it*. She owns the messy, the inconsistent, the colours and the textures that make up her message, her actions, her values, her passions and her voice.

She owns it because she owns herself. And she could only move into ownership once she'd nurtured the seeds of permission.

Women often ask me what the secret to confidence is and my response is always: *ownership*. When you experience a woman who's confidence is emanating, she's in full ownership in that moment.

How ownership works

Ownership is fronting up to all that makes you, *you*. It follows permission because permission states: *I will allow myself to become this way or to do this thing*. Ownership is the action on this permission, the follow through. It uses your body, your voice, your money, your effort and your time.

Ownership is very present, very now, and its Zen nature means it isn't holding fast to something permanently or attached with an iron grip.

All ownership cares about is what you own about yourself

and can embody in this very moment of your life. It wants you to tap into your power – that's its MO.

Ownership uses the *I* word – liberally

Ownership gravitates towards the power of *I*.

I know it can be daunting to start a sentence with this one little letter because it's as if there is no taking it back once it's out there. When we use the word *I*, we are attaching ourselves to an idea, an opinion, an experience, a preference or a personality trait.

You may use the word *you* a lot when you really mean to say *I*. You do this because you are trying to create a sense of community with the person you are speaking with. There's a natural calling inside of you to create connection.

This is often how it goes: *You know when you try to say something to someone and you just can't because you're worried they're going to feel rejection and you don't want that to happen so you stay quiet....do you know what I mean?*

The subtext is: I want to make sure I'm not speaking out of turn, that I don't offend, and that I don't appear different because what I'm saying is too full of emotion to actually speak out about.

When you are on the receiving end of this dialogue, you may feel subtly influenced or even coerced. As soon as someone says: *do you know what I mean?* we're hardwired to nod our heads in the affirmative.

Because we might know what they mean.

Then again, we might not.

When you start using language that has a viewpoint and an opinion, you're actively encouraging ownership. It will tap into confidence and confidence in life increases confidence in sex. The difference between:

you know when you feel like this

and saying

I feel like this, I feel disempowered, I feel hurt, I feel sad

is ENORMOUS.

The proof, of the power of this shift, is in how challenging it is for people to use the word *I*. When you use the word *I* to aptly describe an internal feeling or a sensation or an experience that you've had, you aren't being egotistical.

You're not being selfish. You're not being narcissistic.

What's actually happening is that you're clearly dictating and sharing your experience with someone else. When we own something our body knows the difference and it's better primed to release the story attached to that feeling. From that point, we can move on and move through from skirting around the edges of our power to actually being in our power.

Ownership builds with certain terms

Language truly is a gateway to ownership. I started to fully own this when I kept hearing the sound of my own voice in mid 2017. Now, I wasn't just hearing, but truly listening to, how I was speaking to myself and others. I'd become comfortable with the *I* but for every bit of certainty that the word *I* provided, I ended up diluting it with using words like *might, have to* and *should* over and over. *Might* was becoming my go-to concept for the safety it provided me with. I never really had to commit or be accountable with *might* and I used it a little too liberally, like I was constantly darting the follow-through of my actions. When I think of it, my reason for using *might* was to be honourable. I didn't want to disappoint anyone in case the plans changed or I changed my mind. I knew it was a habit I needed to shake when I wasn't owning what I was doing when I was in my own company, talking to myself by saying things like: *I might just get the butter out of the fridge or I might go to the café and then pop into the shops.* It was chronic. I was using *might* even when I knew I was definitely going to do something. I could only change this habit when I noticed how out of alignment it had me feel.

I traced it back to the shadow of the good girl being at play – she was doing what she could to keep following the crowd and people pleasing. She didn't want to speak out of turn.

It would be a stretch to say that I completely dropped the word might (because I didn't). What I did was noticed when I used might and instead replaced it with *can* and *will.* When I was using the more confident language of ownership, I felt less scatty and more certain. It signified a choice to commit over honouring an obligation or a role that I was pressuring myself to fulfill.

Ownership gave me the power of focus. I could move through life with more certainty when I said one thing and stuck to it, without softening it with reasons and fluff to lessen the blow.

Does any of that feel familiar?

How often do you wish that you could just say a clear *no, I can't,* to something but instead you use the word *maybe* or *I'll have to see?*

I know it well – those times when I have dodged saying no upfront only then to be faced with the ongoing stress of needing to backpedal out of that situation. So while it saved me some anxiety in the moment, being unclear upfront often created a more problematic situation later on. It's a reminder to go back to basics.

Studying safe, consensual human interactions taught me that:

No is a no
Yes is a yes and
Maybe is a no.

You see, I used to think that a *maybe* had a whole lot of *yes*. But *maybe* is not a full *yes*. When I feel it in my own body, it says that there is hesitation, restraint, holding back and that the idea that's been proposed to me isn't something that I'm fully on board with. If I feel that a *maybe* wants to arise from my throat, it means that there's a *no* there.

Experimenting with my *yes* and *no* over time has shown me that, I'm now not only more comfortable with saying my *yes* and *no* but, I have a much more sensitive radar to my body's response. My *no* comes through as a 'I just got kicked in the guts feeling' or the deflated feeling of being overwhelmed – my head becomes scrambled. My *yes* comes through as flushed cheeks, a tingly pelvis and this feeling of being lifted up through my solar plexus. Sometimes I get goosebumps. Sometimes I need to wee!

The more I own my body's responses, and use them like the nuggets of gold that they are, the better able I am to create clear verbal responses that match them.

Ownership asks that you feel the pain first (fully) so that the pleasure can follow

There is a tendency to minimise what we say and feel. Please don't.

I believe when you acknowledge what you feel in the present moment that you have a better chance of processing it and clearing it. Blocks in our bodies are built upon what we haven't allowed ourselves to express, so if it hurts and you don't want to feel it anymore, just go there when it is safe to do so. Cry, scream, mewl, whinge, sob: do anything to get it out rather than swallowing it down to deal with later.

Your feelings are valid.

What helps give ownership really solid ground is speaking to experiences and memories as they are happening. Put a voice to them and relay all of that pain whether you feel safest to do that with a confidante, in therapy, into a voice recording, or through creative pursuits.

I've needed to do this over and over to clear out the crap before sex. Sometimes, Ed and I will get started and I just can't keep going with full presence until I have cleared whatever is bugging me…niggling at me. I have to say it. And when I do, I often cry. And when I cry, I feel better. Clearer. Then, if my body says *yes*, we resume and if an orgasm follows, it works like a little bit of extra releasing and softening. That orgasm becomes medicine that gently brings me down from being uppity to being in ownership of my feelings.

When we start sharing – *this is where I feel rejection, this is where I feel shame…*finish your statement at the point where you have completed your expression of your pain. Full stop.

Resist the temptation to add *but others have it worse* or *but I am grateful for X*. When you have said that in its entirety, the gratitude, the generosity and the flow of deep self-respect and love will come later.

It's a struggle to own all the parts of you when they're jumbled together. Reluctance to own all the negative parts and shadows might well follow you into the bedroom when you feel most vulnerable. What has been kept in a box will suddenly want out at the most inopportune time.

Own the shadows as they are cast and the light will have the chance to illuminate you.

Your libido is your responsibility

Did you know that you are the sole owner of your libido, sexuality and erotic power? That all of *that* is actually in your hands?

That, when it comes to your preferences, likes and dislikes, in sex no one else can answer for you?

Whenever you are asked the age-old bedroom question, "*what do you like?*", you have the chance to step forward into the power of ownership. But rather than simply deflect the attention that comes with that question, by saying "*mmm what do you like?*", nuzzle down into these truths.

It's your responsibility to bring your libido out.
It's your responsibility to give you a green light to be sexual.
It's your responsibility to generate pleasure for you.

One of the main blocks to ownership occurs when the shadow side to the female libido is being passive, and it happens when we feel like it's all too hard, the frustration all too unbearable, and we secretly wish we never had to have sex again (Nooooo, walk back towards the light!)

Your libido is active. It wants you to befriend it and move with it. Your libido knows there's a difference between choosing to be still in sex, and being flat out stuck. Your libido also knows there's a difference between making a move to coax your arousal out and doing something because you think it'll look good on the outside.

The best definition of libido I have ever read was within the pages of Alisa Vitti's book, *WomanCode*:

> **Our libido is the ability to give and receive pleasure, enjoyment and acknowledgment.**

Pleasure, enjoyment and acknowledgment are the foundations of your libido, your mojo, your life force and your sexual energy – whatever it is that you want to call it.

Your libido isn't solely a sexual entity.

Your libido is how comfortable you are with other women, how comfortable you are with pleasure and how you receive a compliment or a gift. It moves into the sexual realm when you examine how curious you are and interested in your sexual expression. Your libido is wearing colours other than black. Your libido is being generous with your heart. Your libido understands that you can change your mind but when it speaks it's certain of what it says.

Your libido isn't who you are in sex.

It isn't what you do in sex.

It's your ability to give and receive pleasure, enjoyment and acknowledgment in all of the facets of your life. Own all of this and you will turn your libido on in a way that only you can.

#2 ALIGNMENT

When you own all your parts, shadows, strengths and quirks there's a much bigger likelihood that the way you show up in the world and the bedroom will be aligned.

Alignment is the immensely sexy, yet very underrated, process of the outside of your life matching and reflecting what lives inside of you.

Possibly the biggest threat to you living your life in alignment right now is societal conditioning, as conditioning depends on us being incongruent. This mismatch happens when we've felt one thing on the inside but have ended up doing something completely different on the outside, usually to people please or to conform to the status quo. Incongruence makes it really hard to feel good about where our life is at and where it's going, since everything feels so out of alignment.

Living in alignment as a woman is what gives societal conditioning the big middle finger. Sometimes, the quietest middle finger is the most powerful.

Alignment brings a quiet power

I've observed that the more we're in alignment in our lives as women, the less we have to talk things up or talk things down. When debriefing with our friends, there's less to unpack and deconstruct in deep conversation because we aren't constantly deliberating about our identity or mulling over the latest drama. We reach this point where we become used to knowing when life is aligned with us and when it isn't.

When we say we want to eat differently, we line up the actions to match that intention.

When we observe that there's a commitment in our life that drains us, rather than lifts us up, we say goodbye to it.

When we say *yes* to our partners desire to have sex, we say *yes* because we want to.

Seeing alignment as sexy has called for me to undo the conditioning that stems mostly from the storylines of films and shows I watched over and over again in my late teens and early twenties. These stories centred around how undesirable it was when the heroine was living out of alignment (usually single), then going on to clean up her act, until finally a partner swooped in to complete her. The clincher of this storyline is that it's only when she gets a partner that she is then seen to be aligned and at her most powerful.

Gradually, the appeal of this limited take on women's stories is giving way to stories that are truly empowering. More women, myself included, are using the energy of our money and time to say that we want to watch women who show up in the world consistently and with integrity. Women who demonstrate alignment from the outset by being the heroine of her own life. These are now my favourite stories.

Learning through these real world stories allows alignment to shine. The desire to live our life in alignment allows us to curb the possibility of leaving this life saying what so many women before us have...*I wish I had, I wish I did, I wish I tried...*

At the heart of it, alignment grants us the peace that we have lived our lives to our fullest potential. Now, living to our fullest potential is personal. Deeply personal. This isn't just about your paid work in the world, it's about how all of the pieces of life integrate for you to become...you. Much like your sex life, living to your fullest potential by living in alignment is completely unique and means you:

...travel solo when you want to be unencumbered and free to make your own decisions

...become a stay at home mum because home is exactly where you want to be

...choose to wear the clothes that suit your body and reflect your personality

...run a community organisation because it mirrors your values

...say *no* to the draining family commitment that you have long outgrown

Giving myself permission to live in alignment has been a series of small, and not so small, personal decisions that has granted me my own liberation and personal health. I'm talking where I live, how I parent, who I'm friends with, how I move, what I purchase, who I pay to help me, how I spend my time in leisure and how I live with my menstrual cycle.

Honestly, living in sync with my menstrual cycle is what has really shown me the power of alignment (and if you don't have a menstrual cycle then I recommend using the lunar or astrological cycles instead). When I factor in where I'm at in my cycle and where my strengths and vulnerabilities lie, I'm empowered to then choose the action to match the feeling. Sometimes it doesn't correspond but, for the most part, I know that the compass of my cycle will guide me to match high intensity training with ovulation and slow and gentle movement with menstruation, or the joy of decluttering in the luteal phase and the mojo to learn new things in the follicular phase.

Alignment is what gave me permission to say goodbye to hormonal contraception forever as a 23-year-old.

Alignment is what gives me permission to choose my actions to match my internal state and feelings as opposed to pretending that I am the same every day.

Alignment is what grants me the permission to be a woman who runs a business with heart and soul for the silent, rather than one that ticks the boxes for the vocal masses.

Alignment is what has me saying goodbye to alcohol for big chunks of time because...it just doesn't feel aligned with me anymore.

And they are the only words you need.

That just doesn't feel aligned with me anymore.

Oh but this does...this feels really aligned with me right now.

By far, the biggest step in alignment I've ever taken was the moment that I stopped trying to make my offering to women be about what everyone else thought my message *should* be. When I owned that my clients weren't coming to see me for sizzling hot bedroom romps and oral sex tips, but to unravel the conditioning and trauma that's blocking their capacity to open up, it was like I had given myself permission to keep my eyes completely on my own lane.

Once I took a very long look inward at what kind of sex life I have and how I show up in this world and owned that part, I could actually hear the *click, click, click* of the parts coming together. From that moment on, I could live in alignment because I didn't have to strive in my sex life to have all the answers for the clients I wasn't even actually serving. I could serve women with such quiet power because I knew them through knowing me.

Listen for the *click, click, click* in your own life and you know alignment has come to grace you.

#3 SOVEREIGNTY

Permission is fundamental to liberation.

You're free when you live as you choose.

You're free when you have fire in your loins and the way you express that fire is true for you.

You're free when you live your life from a place of wholehearted giving to yourself and giving to others without the constant self-sacrifice, martyr mode and burnout. You're free when your lover holds you in their arms and you are completely at peace with the possibility of sex being propositioned. You experience sex as an act of co-creation.

In digging deep for the gold, I realised that there was a vital trait that bridges permission and liberation.

Sovereignty.

Sovereignty is a classic political term that I reconceptualise as a personal movement. A true permission granter is a sovereign being. Drawing upon the political definition, she has the full right and power of a governing body over herself. She is autonomous as she moves through life abandoning the notion of *I have to* and choosing instead the motto *I want to*.

You are the heroine

Sovereignty means that you'll be a lone ranger(ette) at times. Rather than look outward to who you can impress, it requires a good, solid dose of ruffling your own feathers. When you are the true heroine of your sex life, you don't depend on another person to validate you. You aren't waiting to be rescued because you step up for yourself.

Do what you want to do in life, and sex, because it ruffles your own feathers.

Do it because it's exhilarating to keep growing.

Do it because you are your only competition in this life.

The beauty of sovereignty is that you can be in something on your own, with others alongside you in the wings helping, cheering and supporting.

Although being sovereign may look isolating, it's not the same as it would be if you were to fly solo, or to not give a shit about what others think or feel. The sovereign woman isn't aloof, disconnected or frankly, a bitch. If anything, a woman in her sovereignty is better posed to trust other people because she trusts herself. The power of her autonomy stems from the ability to simultaneously rely on herself with complete certainty while she chooses occasions to collaborate with others.

When I picture a woman in her sovereignty, I see her as magnetic, untouchable, radiant, certain and assured.

The women I look to as sovereign have some common threads. Rather than being needy for attention by over-sharing, she will tell her story with a gentle cadence. I instantly feel that she isn't doing this to boast about her achievements, but because the listener will learn from her clarity.

In her maturity, she tells it like it is. Her ability to strike the fine balance of being full of emotion without the need for consoling, or sympathy, from strangers and friends, is the ultimate display of personal health. Her struggles aren't for the public to devour as gossip.

It's easy to get jealous of how the sovereign woman makes hard work look…well, easy. Stepping up to the plate again and again is old hat for her, yet she never bitches about it and she never forgets her roots. Never assume she's had it easy. Instead, know that she has crafted her life in this graceful way because of the hard path she has had to walk. I believe sovereign women are gifted a heavy load, heavier than many of us could carry, because she can handle it.

The sovereign woman is up for bearing this heaviness because life knows that she is capable. More than capable.

In everyday life though, the sovereign woman is:

- the work colleague that gets her work done autonomously and approaches you for your valuable input. She does this to invite in an alternate viewpoint, not to be validated.

- the woman that self-pleasures with satisfaction and can hold her own in sex with another by speaking up and following her body's lead.

- the devoted partner that can happily spend time alone in her own company and will ask you at a later time if there is something you want to do together. She does this to forge connection not as a distraction from the restlessness of her own company.

- the friend that you don't hear from for a while and suddenly calls. She does this because she prefers to have clear space to listen and share with you not because a date on a calendar says it's time to catch up again.

- the ever-present mama that's in tune with her child's needs and knows when healthy separation is necessary. She does this to become closer to her child through the opportunity to nurture herself not because she is selfish or doesn't enjoy them.

When I speak to these examples, I'm speaking of myself. I'm speaking of the women that have been permission granters for me. They have showed me the moments when we can choose acts of self-respect and integrity over acts of fear and desperation.

Sovereignty, for me, has meant that despite countless requests for my services to be available through Medicare and private health insurance, I have purposefully avoided this route in favour of being uncensored, autonomous and outspoken. Becoming part of a bigger system would have meant ticking a lot of boxes to ensure that I conformed to a set of ideals that I don't necessarily hold myself. After being a nurse in a very big health system for 15 years, I had zero desire to recreate that sense of powerlessness.

My need to be sovereign may have cost me financially, but I am being repaid in all facets of my life with alignment, ownership, confidence and the sweetness of liberation.

When I'm in sovereignty, I feel both empowered, and in my power. On the inside, even when I'm in doing mode and being active, everything is effortless. Sovereignty's grace and purity comes from the truth that you simply couldn't live in any other state. None of this is for show or the gratification of others. Moving through life this way taps directly into our primal knowing that being alone and feeling lonely are two very different states.

The challenges of being your own permission granter

Being your own permission granter reaps great rewards through conquering the maze of challenges it throws up. All of this happens to bring you closer to being your real self so if you can edge through these testing experiences, you'll be all the more fully *you* on the other side. Some of these feelings may never go away so I reckon we might as well get comfortable with them so that we can face them a little more objectively.

Guilt

Before you become your own permission granter, it's pretty likely that you are going to feel some guilt around it.

Guilt arises when you feel as though you've compromised your own standards of conduct or violated a universal standard, which is often an unwritten law. Could I ask that you pay attention to the words, *when you feel as though*? When you feel guilt, is it your guilt or is it the feeling that you should be guilty based on what other people would think?

Permission granting allows you to come into who you are meant to be and that can make other people uncomfortable. As you fully form and start to own all your pieces, the guilt that you feel won't necessarily be about your own standards, but everyone else's standards that you've internalised. Guilt is that part of you that always worries how your true and aligned actions will affect others, and guilt will work tirelessly to try and keep your big dreams in lockdown. It will show up to derail all the efforts you have made, which remind me of those persistent thoughts of giving up during the transition phase of birth. In this phase of my own birth experiences, I wanted to give up so badly. With the same bloody music on repeat and a cold washcloth on my head, I was fantasising about swapping lives with my midwife or frankly, anyone who walked in the room. If I had been given the chance to not be in the discomfort of my own body and experience I would have taken it. What started off strong; a knowing of exactly where I was going with getting those babies into my arms safely, morphed into a yearning to be wheeled out of the warmth of the birth suite and into theatre. My spirit was tired and I had no idea of how I was going to finish what I started. Fear was setting in and fear inhibits labour.

After having my first baby, I was let in on a little secret. The transition phase is normal. I didn't know that the feeling that I had actually has a name and it's notorious not just for being when you want to give up but when the biggest part of your progress is just around the corner.

I feel the same way about guilt. If you can move through the 'guilt transition phase' on your way to becoming your own permission granter, then it's possible that the best part is yet to come. Don't let the guilt stop your progress. There's something much more important that wants to be birthed by you.

In those times guilt comes up, remember that guilt is reminding you of your tendency to serve and protect the feelings of others before yourself. Take a moment to consider what the cost is for you if you don't take these steps towards becoming your own permission granter.

When I feel tempted to let guilt and some old script about what women, wives and mothers *should* be, I need only think of how my liberation will pave the way and create a ripple effect for so many other women – women I don't even know. On the home front, I think about how my two girls are witnessing their mama live as her own permission granter and all the guilt instantly melts away. Trust that your empowerment will empower others and that is nothing to feel guilty about.

Imposter Syndrome

As you move through the guilt (or feel the guilt and do it anyway), there may also be a period of calibration as you create your own blueprint of permission granting. The awkwardness and uncertainty that comes with calibration can mean that you imitate others in order to find yourself.

From saying a throwaway line that you heard another woman say, to becoming a flat out carbon copy, a little bit of imposter syndrome will probably happen at some point. When you notice a bit of wannabe show up in you, take pause to ask if what you're doing is actually in alignment with you. As you absorb the wisdom and green lights of others, trust that with time, you'll become clearer on the occasions where you are taking aspects from another person because they are aligned with you, and the times where you're lost and need a bit of fake it 'til you become it.

The more I have persisted in honing in on my own voice and stance in this world, the less I feel like an imposter. Maybe it played out this way because I didn't stop searching at the point where I was more dependent on other women who shone a light on what was possible for me. With my neck cranked against the ceiling of trying to second guess what my next move should be, I eventually got tired. I could either, fall back down, quit and walk back into an easy life, or break through the imposter ceiling, hold tight and catapult through to become me.

Rejection

When you're a self-sourcing permission granter living as sovereign, you run the risk of rejection. Stay the course. Persistence will pay you back generously.

You see, sovereignty, ownership, alignment and permission are all intertwined and to be sure, you'll be tested. I've been tested. In permission granting's most testing times, the only drum beating I can hear is my own. My life can sound like an echo chamber as my own voice continuously vibrates the walls of my existence. I often find myself living as if there's no proof as to why I am creating my life in this way. The mission of raising the volume on one of society's most taboo topics has left me hearing nothing but white noise for months, sometimes even years at a time.

There have been moments where I'm holding my breath for something that has the promise of cracking me open, only to have it fizzle out before me. Rejection is a feeling I know well.

In mid 2017 the possibility of a partnership in my home city, that could have given me a lot more reach to women who suffer in silence, came tumbling down quickly. It took a little while for me to say 'fuck it' with honesty. On my birthday in October, I vividly recall standing in the kitchen with a glass of champagne and spontaneously sobbing to friends about how it was just another sign that I don't belong anywhere. Those were the exact words I cried, completely exasperated: *I just don't belong anywhere.*

Rejection became a flavour I tasted daily. My work liberating women didn't fit inside an already established box and, I got much later on that, this can be really triggering for a lot of people. In my case, it was triggering to the people who will never actually be clients of mine. Older male medical professionals effectively barricaded me from helping women that probably wouldn't be triggered by the message of female empowerment. It was a hard one to move on from. I decided that I couldn't let the rejection from men stop me from reaching women.

Fast forward to 2018, and I'm actually thankful that the partnership didn't eventuate. Turns out there was this strange little moment that happened when I was in talks where my gut punched me and said 'you will have to censor yourself to be connected to this organisation' and I told my body: *Be quiet. I'll work all of that out later. It's OK to bend a little with my own voice because it will mean more business growth.* The fact that I remember that split second in time says to me that the message from my gut was loud in volume and truth. My gut knew I would have been censored and controlled and that would have blocked me from exploring my ownership, alignment and sovereignty. As always, my gut was right.

Moments like the one above, where I have to feel the full spectrum of guilt, imposter syndrome and rejection, are when being my own permission granter can get really frustrating, and I get tempted to fall back into some sort of easy-going, normal-ish life.

When trust feels so far away, I remind myself that easy is not a challenge. After being sovereign for a few years, the very notion of following the pack makes me restless and jolts me into a defence of *but I know better than them* mode. The truth is, I don't actually know better than them, but I definitely know myself, and my perspective, better than them. Easy is fun, and a nice place to visit once in a while, but I wouldn't want to stay there forever.

Being my own permission granter asked me to reach and live beyond easy. Being liberated, to me, means having my eyes wide open so that I can dodge being duped. I can walk through life with my head held high knowing that I'm always acting within my own best interests and that these parameters give me a sense of freedom.

Personally, it only takes a quick mental foray into adolescence to re-experience all the times I didn't listen to my knowing and chose to trust someone else instead. While I'm willing to heap it all into the pile that is labelled *life experiences*, there's something that gnaws at me when I think about how this distrust of my own green light followed me into adulthood. Although it was subtler than adolescence, it was still rooted in the same problem.

I didn't trust myself so
I didn't explore my body so
I didn't work out what I liked because it was too hard and
I wanted someone else to work it out for me and
I needed the presence of a guy to validate me

All of these short cuts took me a very long way from myself. Sure, I could live like this – my life wasn't going to be taken from me if I went through every day seeking validation and using that to sustain my identity. But was that what I wanted my life to be?

It was a slow, slow, transition in coming to realise that the anxiety of having to tick the boxes was actually taking my real life from me, so I began to shift just one aspect at a time. If you could watch the montage, you would see me wading into the waters to tweak one aspect of my life at a time. In other words, it was the longest montage ever.

I started to live by my own rules when I got that I'd lost touch with my essence as a woman, which is being sovereign and radiant. In my neediness – scrambling for a validity hit, I wasn't able to be present with the maturity of being part of a collective with other women. My focus was all on asking that they tell me what to do and not really listening to what it was that they had to share with me.

It's OK that it played out that way. Perhaps I had to go through an era of disempowerment and external permission granting to come even closer to the truth that my sovereignty is a treasure that isn't guaranteed by life conditions…that I can be threatened not only by what is outside of me, but also by what is inside of me. And that although permission granting is my birth right, I can still be at risk of losing my way with it when I'm scared about the ramifications of rejection and abandonment.

Permission granting is my advantage.

It's your advantage. It's our secret sauce to being exactly who we want to be in sex and life. Until we all really follow that invitation, we'll continue to feel stifled, numb and anything but libidinous.

And to be libidinous is to be alive.

The permission pledge

Moving out of the habit to look to others to explain your sexuality to you is scary terrain. When you want to shut down, keep the focus on how permission, and the golden trifecta that fuels it, is moving you forward, edging you closer to your liberation.

Your liberation means that you are living in your own personal version of health.

When you feel like you are closing in, this is what you need to pledge to yourself.

With one hand on your heart and one hand on your womb space or pussy, use your throat to say:

I pledge that I will give myself permission to own all the parts, facets, nooks and crannies of my body and my identity.

When it comes to my libido, I own it.

I pledge that I will give myself permission to dance the dance of alignment in my life.

When it comes to my libido, I am in alignment.

I pledge that I will give myself permission to be sovereign and know that this is the secret to my radiance.

When it comes to my libido, I am sovereign.

TWO

The Good Girl

HEY, COME IN A LITTLE CLOSER.

A little closer again.

I'm speaking in hushed tones because I want your good girl to hear this.

Before we move into exactly what you need permission for in your sex life, we need to talk about the good girl persona, and how it inhabits so many of us in our daily life.

No doubt she'll be with you throughout this whole personal introspection thing.

That's because she's always been with you and there's a really good chance she will always be with you. Imprinted and ingrained into your fibres.

If you aren't quite sure of who your good girl is, (aside from an adult affirming that you were a 'good girl' growing up), then this is your chance to get closer to a key part of who is driving you. In knowing and owning your good girl, you're given a very important green light to step into your own personal liberation, simply because you understand how she works for you and how she limits your truest expression.

Sexologists are good girls too

I like to think I know how to navigate my good girl well, but sitting down to write this, I'm shown so vividly how dominating she still is and how urgent she can be. She's an impatient bugger! I'm often still left dumbfounded at the times she shows up unannounced. You'd think that I would've gotten a really good grip on how to tame her by now but she can be activated by the most innocuous circumstances – usually when I'm speaking with someone who I perceive to be an authority or an elder. Sometimes I get a choice to call her out, oftentimes I don't realise she's inhabiting me until I blink and realise *Oh! She's here!*

In forging my own path of personal and sexual liberation, I've come to know my good girl exceedingly well. Yes she's part of me, but she isn't *all* of me.

You'll soon notice that I speak of my good girl as a *she* because she is one of my many parts. I'm purposefully not using the term *I* to speak about these traits and behaviours of mine because they so often come together to make up what I now know as my good girl. She's one of my masks, one of my identities, one of my archetypes inside of me that I call on. And like any mask, identity or archetype, she is comprised of light and shade.

In learning how to give ourselves permission, we need to own all of how our good girl helps and hinders our growth into the more elusive waters of womanhood.

When my clients are embodying their good girl, they commonly express concern that I might not be able to help them because they fear that they are experiencing an isolated human experience.

The good girl in torment is always worried that she's alone as a good girl in torment. It's as if she has come to expect that her predicament of high-achievement and the numbness that goes with that is unique. This isn't to say *you* aren't unique (because you are) but your problem isn't.

I promise, as a good girl you're never alone.

There's an army of good girls out there who are living in complete disconnection from their personal liberation because it's scary and *feels* so unknown to them (emphasis on the *feels*). She's never dared to investigate or probe what lies inside of her for fear of opening the lid on a bottomless well of feelings that she has worked really hard to compartmentalise and control.

The following is how I've seen and felt the good girl both within my clients and myself. I've noticed that she thrives off of certain conditions and has specific priorities.

Reading through, you gotta love and admire the good girl's focus on what she deems important. Her tenacity is unparalleled.

Striving and Achieving

I'll be straight up honest. I love my inner good girl because she gets shit done. If she says that she's going to do something, she'll do it, especially if other people are depending on her.

My inner good girl is the part of me that wants to strive, yearns to achieve, and above all wants to ensure that everyone is pleased with what they see, and what they feel, when it comes to my actions and my way of life.

Is my good girl a people pleaser? Yup.

My good girl has serious drive and fire and is the part of me that says: *keep showing up and doing your best.* The only problem with that is that she can sometimes be wilful. Her dogged determination finds it easy to ignore and disregard the power of her gut instincts.

When I silence my gut, I end up pushing through, even when I'm exhausted and need rest, whether it be my work, tending to my home or the must-do tasks, my good girl mindset will say: *just one more thing, just one more thing* as if there will never be one more thing. She traps me into believing that when this one more thing is done, then I can rest. When all the things are done, then and only then am I worthy of enjoying the fruits of life that are slow and purposeless.

I secretly call her a taskmaster.

The taskmaster mode comes with another shadow. She not so secretly has a thing for self-flagellation. She can see that something is 99% done but she'll pour all her focus on the 1% that isn't done in her mind. What she values most is a sense of completion because then she'll be rewarded. This shadow has required extensive untangling on my part as I've come to rely upon acknowledging and rewarding myself first instead of automatically going to get it from other people.

My inner good girl doesn't want to cause a fuss. She doesn't want to stir things up because she likes to keep the peace. Thinking about it now, it seems so bizarre that this place of external peace is what she seeks when she is anything but peaceful on the inside. She's always a flurry with activity and the anxiety of not being and doing enough. There's something to be said for the old saying I learnt working in mental health: *External order. Internal chaos.* This sums up what really lies underneath the good girl in torment. The outside looks so calm, poised and collected but the inside is clamouring for release.

In the strangest twist, her being outwardly meek and amiable is what makes her dangerous.

The good girl has so many admirable traits that it can be hard to see how she could misstep when it comes to moving her way through life. Whether it be applying for a job, organising a catch-up, getting taxes done, buying a secure property, pushing through a high intensity workout, nudging kids out the door, researching a new way of eating or de-cluttering a room, you will want her there (actually, she will show up anyway because that's what she does).

But turn down the lights, hold her hands and motion for her to come sit next to you on the bed, and you may start to see her flip out. She malfunctions because intimacy is vague, feeling is fleeting and uncontrollable, and sex is a messy, heart opening, pleasure fuelled tryst without purpose. Her checklist just can't factor it all in and that has her feeling threatened.

Throughout *Permission*, you will come to see how she can still be with you in those moments where she feels so out of place. We don't want her gone; we want her right there with us because she belongs.

Social conformity

My good girl has a front that prioritises keeping within certain social bounds and norms. She likes to be, just comfortably, in the middle of this invisible spectrum so as not to draw any attention to her perceived flaws. When she mingles, she aims to be neither too much nor not enough. She despises being socially awkward or politically incorrect.

My inner good girl is the part of me that seeks validation, that seeks reassurance and that always wants to know: *did I do this right?*, as if there is some universal standard of what is right. She does this with tact. She does everything with tact as she is ever-mindful of how she comes across.

When I'm in my good girl mode, I have power blinkers on. It isn't until after I've walked away from an interaction that I realise how much of my power I swallowed down, all because of the need to be seen a certain way.

My good girl doesn't want to ruffle feathers.

My good girl doesn't want to draw attention to herself, unless it's because she has achieved something truly remarkable. She will do anything to avoid bad press, being the fodder of gossip, or being spoken ill of.

Even as a fully-fledged woman, my good girl gets distressed when getting caught out by certain family members having a puff of a ciggie once a year (or so. Who's counting?). That sideways glance of disapproval stays with her long after the festivities are over.

And that is the crux of what tears women apart internally – the pull to preserve a persona, whilst being true and genuine in the present moment.

Risk aversion

My good girl likes to avoid risks wherever possible. The anxiety of keeping everything within certain parameters means that she expects certain outcomes. Risk is way too risky because she doesn't believe she can navigate through the waters of uncertainty. Although she's used to living in anticipation, it pains her when the anticipation is closely followed by disappointment and, even worse, a loose end that isn't neatly tied up.

I'll confess my inner good girl was so tested by transitioning from a very secure day job with super superannuation, benefits, and a regular pay cheque, to living firmly within the world of entrepreneurship. Her need to anticipate what comes next and what everything is going to look like meant a lot of trepidation moving through some very uncertain waters.

So I looked inward and asked my good girl:

'Were you happy in your secure day job?'

'No. But I knew what to expect and I like that'

'Would you prefer to know what to expect or to live in a way where you feel free and aligned as a woman?'

'I'm still tempted to say go back to the day job because I don't like risk. But then I think – what if the risk is worth it? What if the risk has security beyond my wildest dreams but it's just the transition phase that's hard?'

Yes. What if?

I've learnt that when I keep my good girl filled in on all the facts, I can be in a lengthy, engaged dialogue with her. When I stopped and reduced it down to what her core strengths and insights are, I realised that she's just looking out for me and I love her fiercely for that.

Neat and organised

When women come to see me and share their sexual story, they are usually dressed and presented as impeccably as their means can afford. The good girl persona likes to be well presented and neat. In fact, neat is one of her favourite things in life, along with organised. Neat and organised.

She likes her schedule and her list of things that she can tick off because then she knows where she stands. Work and life often meld because she likes the sense of achievement in both of these realms.

My inner good girl loves to learn so that she can keep moving towards this place of assurance that doesn't actually exist. When in full flight, she believes there's this magical final destination where she will feel satiated, but she hasn't quite worked out yet, that she will never actually arrive. However, my body knows this and sends up a warning flare to inform me that some of these endeavours to learn more are fruitless and will never bring satisfaction. In fact, they often sap me of the energy I need to live my real, heartfelt, life.

Thinking beats feeling

When the good girl is switched on she'll answer the question *how do you feel?* immediately with the words *I think...* The good girl is so accustomed to having her very snug thinking hat on that she struggles to take it off. That's OK, this is just a habit at play. It can take time to learn to listen to the whispers of your heart and intuition when you're used to working with your head and all of the *shoulds* in your life.

At her most cerebral, the good girl likes precision. She likes words like *correct, perfect* and *exactly* because there's no room for movement, and if there's no room for movement, she knows where she stands.

She loathes telling stories about her own life, especially when she doesn't think she has any stories. Other times in conversation, you feel like you can actually witness her discomfort as she passes the baton back to the person she's in conversation with. That discomfort arises when she doesn't want personal attention. This isn't an issue if the topic at hand is heady in nature, but when it comes to what it is she feels and topics she considers vulnerable, she just wants to cower away. All of *that* is in a box, and one harmless conversation can threaten to tarnish the veneer.

Her capacity to be selective about what she reveals to the world is an important and admirable trait. But the setback shows up when she finds someone she loves and struggles to open up. This happens when the good girl mask is still on in the bedroom and, despite her efforts to drop the mask and step into womanhood, her feet and her spirit remain, firmly, planted where they are. She's just so used to having her good girl call the shots that any part of her that craves raw intimacy goes unexpressed.

She thinks her way through sex in order to protect herself.

What the good girl really needs is permission for her feelings to come out and play.

A rigid body

One of the first things I notice when a woman is sitting before me, wanting to be seen as 'good', is that her body is rigid in the chair. I say this regardless of her body's shape and size and how nervous she is about coming and talking about her sex life. Holding her body a certain way is an old pattern that dies hard when the good girl is in full effect. Her body likes to be exact and upright because she doesn't know how to relax, soften and just sink down. I've had countless women share with me that even sitting on the couch at home, she is stiff and locked, as though she is a flower that can never unfurl.

Once we've identified that sense of being locked in her body, we make simple movements together to unlock and access other identities within her.

Permission to move out of good girl mode, even for a few moments, starts with putting your feet on the floor, opening your palms, allowing your pelvis to rock back and, most importantly, switching your core muscles OFF for a while. I've observed that living in good girl mode often means protecting your power centre in your solar plexus around your belly button. It's as if your abdominals believe that if they stay on guard then you can keep all of your power in and at bay.

Learning to embrace womanhood and feeling a sense of release means allowing our tummies to be soft. It's safe for the good girl to be soft.

This little hack also has a bonus effect of turning your pelvic floor muscles off and allowing them to rest, which is much needed respite for those who feel tightness with penetration and pain with sex.

Ignoring our good girl can turn the volume up on her shadow side, in that she becomes more rigid and more perfectionistic.

I propose living life *with* her rather than against her, by allowing her the space to be purposeful and satiated. You might need to give your good girl permission to be present and to be there.

I wrote this love letter to my good girl.

Perhaps you would like to write to your good girl too.

She's always seeking your acknowledgment.

A LOVE LETTER TO MY GOOD GIRL

Good girl,

Thank you, thank you and thank me for everything you have done for me. I still need you, I always will. You have been an integral part of my identity, forming and shaping me so that I can be elevated to much higher levels of productivity and output.

I'm just wondering if I could have some moments alone so that you can go and rest. You might not realise that you need to recuperate and take a breath so that I too can have a chance to rest and recuperate. I would love for us to embody a healthy relationship that ebbs and flows, not feels like it is stuck in one gear with one outcome. We tried that and now I'm ready for us to have a new dynamic.

I promise I'll call on you when I need you. You always know how to be kind to a stranger, how to knuckle down and get mundane head tasks done and I love how your keen organisation skills can empower another person to care about having their shit together when life is messy.

Good girl, I give you permission to show up without suffocating me.

I give you permission to fuel my tasks without making tasks my life.

I give you permission to step aside at times where I really need the liberation of being in a state of feeling rather than doing.

I love you and thank you my inner good girl
Thank you +
Thank me

Lauren xo

PART 2

THREE

Permission to be sexual

PERMISSION TO BE SEXUAL doesn't mean you need to take action. Yet. We're in the early stages that simply ask if you can consider the possibility of being sexual. I want to assure you that you don't have to completely believe it and you definitely don't have to go out and prove yourself.

Permission to be sexual is all about harnessing what's already inside of you, tweaking some fixed beliefs to become more flexible and sharpening your capacity to be critical about what triggers you.

Embracing your sexual woman with a healthy attitude means that we're putting the spotlight on what you already are, not what you aren't.

Your sexual foundation needs to be inclusive of your capacity to execute your yes and your no. The past has passed. In the weight of this moment, you're empowered to move ahead with renewed standards. These standards exist for you and for your sexual partners.

Your libido has been conditioned

The safe and natural expression of female sexuality has had such a turbulent past that women aren't required to have a history of abuse or assault to feel sexually disconnected. I believe that we all have sexual trauma and will explore this deeper in the *Permission to have trauma* chapter.

I've had women say to me that they feel guilty about having sexual problems because they have never experienced trauma. I'll say to you now, what I said to them: Trauma and abuse are not the only pre-cursors to sexual shutdown. It's possible to have the vitality of your libido suffocated before it even had the chance to take a full, life giving breath. That, in itself, is a form of betrayal that moves just like trauma.

Disconnection from your sexual nature doesn't always have a clear origin. It can be as straightforward, but as complex, as thousands of different messages and influences telling you, in all sorts of ways, that to be sexual is to be bad. Most women I have worked with have a distinct memory of equating being sexual with being bad, naughty or dirty.

For some, they had the fear of becoming pregnant, and being ostracised, as their motivation to suppress their sexual impulses. For others, the absence of affectionate touch and talk of sex in the household meant that they emerged into adulthood with no idea what to do in the bedroom. Years later, sex is now an awkward, and sometimes painful, way of trying to feel that special kind of intimacy with the person they love.

Conditioning targets all forms of sexual expression. Women who are sexually liberated are shamed in so many ways and it feels even more vicious when it's other women who are instigating the shaming. I loathe saying that women can be the harshest judges of female sexual expression.

Watching the film *Pitch Perfect* a number of years ago felt like another bruise to a very old injury. If you haven't seen it, one of the running jokes amongst *The Bellas,* a cappella singing group, is that group members who have sex with one of the opposing a cappella groups are instantly labelled a *slut* and ousted. This wasn't a stand-alone verbal threat – they actually followed through by kicking their own team members out if they breeched this code. This joke activated a deep wound within me. It's the wound of betrayal, which stings even more when instigated by a sister.

On a wider level, this is a film with far-reaching influence and a very direct message – express yourself sexually with someone we don't approve of and you won't belong. Fear of being banished is a pretty effective way of shutting our legs so closely together that we don't dare misstep.

I've done the time of living with my legs closed shut and
my groin in a constant state of contraction
and it didn't serve me.

I've done the time of running with the
pack to ensure I belong.

I've done the time of trying to live in this impossible
space of not being too much and not being enough.

When I feel into my libido, I just want it to feel liberated.

Traits of the sexual woman

The woman who is at ease with her sexuality is comfortable with being recognised as a sexual woman. I've noticed over the years that there are some common threads amongst the women who are fully merged with their sexual nature. What really stands out to me is how the sexual woman is equally humble and outspoken. She has fire but she doesn't bang on about it all day. You can just feel her heat without naming it.

The following is a composite of what I believe to be a sexual woman. Emulate her where you can – just make sure you keep your own original flavour flowing through because there is no sexual woman quite like you.

She declares herself as a sexual woman

If you want permission to flow in your veins so fervently that it's an inextricable part of your being, then it boils down to declaring this:

I am a sexual woman.

Say it with me.
Say it out LOUD.

When you say it out loud, you activate a truth and being sexual can then move from being a *faraway notion* to being your new normal. When you have the courage to say *I am a sexual woman*, it highlights how much pain fuels the words *I'm just not a sexual person*. Your libido can hear you whether it's merely circulating around your mind or it's something that you say in conversation. More to the point, your libido not only hears you, it listens and it responds accordingly. Rather than act out of rebellion and prove you wrong, it will take you literally and move towards shutdown.

When you say the words *I am a sexual woman*, you're making a declaration. You're allowing all your yearnings to surface – confidence, certainty, clarity, trust, affection and ownership. You bet the most embodied, juicy, sexual, sassy woman you can think of OWNS this part of herself and not only believes it but believes *in* it.

Something I had to ask myself was: how high can your volume go when you squash your potential down?

You are a sexual woman.
I am a sexual woman.

She loves her sexuality more than her sex life

In order to fully blossom into being a sexual woman, it's essential that you love your sexuality more than you love your sex life. Your sexuality is a reflection of you, but your sex life isn't.

I think it's important to distinguish the two so that you know what parts of you need focus and care. Usually, by a long shot, our sexuality needs our focus first.

Your sexuality is your internal feelings and responses about what you perceive to be erotic and sexual in nature. It's malleable and flexible and can't be reduced down to who you are attracted to. I go so far as to say it's how comfortable you are watching a good sex scene, it's how you respond to flirting; it's what stirs you up to feel something delicious, pleasurable (and sometimes forbidden).

Your sexuality is a luscious trigger.

Nothing can explode within your sex life unless your sexuality is in a good place.

Your sexuality is more important than your sex life because it needs to be tended to so that you have a good sex life. Nurture and nourish it with books, conversations, art, film, music and information that support you in being real and bullshit free. You'll know your sexuality is conversing with you when you easily identify the facets of life that have sexual undertones. You'll feel the charge of the erotic create electric sparks as your pupils dilate with arousal and something in your pelvis is woken up. In laywoman's terms, you'll feel horny and turned on.

But feeling horny or turned on doesn't necessarily mean you want to act on these feelings. This is the key difference between permission and consent (your 'yes' or 'no') in action.

I cringe to admit that in the midst of envy my head will sometimes throw up the words *'but it's easy for her'* when I really don't know a woman's whole story. The same goes for the woman who's in love with her sexuality. She doesn't necessarily carry out the following with ease, mostly because she may still feel the discomfort of operating against her habits to be meek, quiet and unseen. Yet, when she honours the full force of her libidinous nature, she:

...embraces the way she holds herself – physically and in her presence

...flirts and smiles with her eyes

...is unapologetic in that she isn't constantly saying sorry for all of the ways she moves through life

...says 'fuck yes' to her body in the mirror (however it looks)

...has a conscious awareness of her desires – especially those that don't require physical expression

...lets herself be taken away by art forms that make her feel the sexual undercurrent of life and above all...

Knows that deep down she's sexual despite her conditioning

Your sex life is what you do with your body and others bodies in a tryst of sexual touch and energy exchange. It's an authentic extension of your sexuality but it isn't ALL of you.

Love your sexuality more than your sex life.

She endorses low quantity, high quality

Just when I think we've all moved on from gauging how good sex is from the amount of times we have it per week, month or year, I have another client walk into my office feeling like she just isn't interested in having sex enough to clock up the frequency to *more*. It's an old story – it's the one that says that being sexual means having more sex. It has taken me years to untangle myself from that one. There's no meter measuring how sexual you are and if there was, it wouldn't be based on quantity.

So when it comes to sex, if you can, drop the notion of *more* for now. Actually, drop it forever. I know your good girl might not like that but dropping more will give her permission to put her over-achieving feet up.

This is the full green light to focus only on quality, regardless of what your partner is focusing on in your sex life.

Being an emboldened sexual woman isn't about how often you have sex.

For me and the women I work with, it's a lot more appealing to have one quality interaction a week or a fortnight than having sex that you are merely tolerating and aren't psyched for several times a week.

The more you say *yes* to sex that doesn't fulfil your needs, the more your body will start to close down. If once a week feels too confronting, feel free to change the frequency to once a fortnight or once a month.

I've seen and written about all sorts of suggestions when it comes to healthy relationships where sexual activity is low and I reckon once a week, somewhere between 30 and 60 minutes is realistic and doable. When you add it all up, 30 minutes a week ends up being just over 24 hours in one year.

I asked myself this question: *Could you spend one day of 365 days giving your sexual life attention, focus, acknowledgment, pleasure and enjoyment?*

If apprehension, avoidance and shutdown have been shadowing your capacity to open in the bedroom then start with a smaller time frame. Most importantly, I often say that something once a week is better than nothing so that you can start to create new sexual memories and have a sense of mastery as you grow. There's so much power in the small in that it comes together to contribute to something long-lasting.

She is self-centred

Being self-centred is vital and the sexual woman knows this. Your sexuality is not a treasure to be given away to placate someone else. Despite what conditioning may have said to women en masse, it isn't selfish to have needs and preferences in sex. When we are operating from a place of selfish, we have a complete disregard for the consequences of our actions on others.

Yet when we are self-centred, we are exactly that – centred in ourselves. Solid and certain. When it comes to your sex life, there has to be something in it for you or you won't have any desire to return to it. So if you're struggling with the physical arousal side of sex, you need to come back to what it is you want to feel in sex.

Your incentive needs to be feelings based before it's sensations based.

This self-centredness and self-assurance that naturally flows through the sexual woman means that she's not always well received. As you allow yourself to become the sexual woman, there will be times where your friendliness will be misinterpreted as flirting and "wanting it" or your confidence is misinterpreted as arrogance. This opening may have you feeling isolated if it's misunderstood. I assure you it's temporary, especially as you come to surround yourself in the company of people who respect you and love you as you are.

In your isolation, you may over-share to the wrong person and feel shame. Or you may over-share and liberate them, you don't always know. Speaking out about sexuality is a gamble. The topics sheer sensitivity and taboo nature often means you don't ask questions because you don't want to pry. The problem is that, years later, we often come to realise the flaw of this approach as we suddenly say: *why didn't I know that? Why didn't anyone tell me?*

Where is the line between being intrusive and being informative? You won't always know. Just promise me you won't let that line keep you permanently quiet.

Her sexuality is private, but her libido is public

The sexual woman keeps her sexuality inside of her and is selective about who touches it. She shares it in the ways that she loves to when it feels right to. Even in times of uncertainty, when she feels alone, and feels that no one can meet her, she keeps the searchlight on for the right person and right conditions. These are both waiting to be found.

I believe that the private nature of your sexuality means that you need to know it before someone else can truly appreciate it and act as a contributor. No one else can weave the threads to make you the masterpiece that you are. You may think another soul will coax your sexiness out of you but deep down only you can.

So if you need to source inspiration for your sexuality, look straight to your libido. That's the part of you that is out there, fronting up in broad daylight. The people that exist around you will already know where your libido is at. As much as you might want to, you can't hide or conceal it.

A high libido raises its eyebrows, smiles and charges forth with enthusiasm and joy.

When your libido is low, it's operating at a sub-optimal level in your daily life. A low libido mumbles and gives a shoulder shrug as a response to what life presents.

Be the woman with the high libido for life and your libido for sex will follow suit.

The easiest way to increase your libido for life is to follow what feels good and to engage with what you truly enjoy. I get how obvious that sounds. But there are just way too many women walking around in depletion, holding tightly to the attitude that life is being done to them. Having a high libido for life means, owning where you have choice and, using your time wisely so you can get juiced up and nourished. These are some of my hacks for having a high libido for life:

- I spontaneously sing and dance in the kitchen
- I forge close relationships with businesses I am loyal to. It feels good to be greeted with acknowledgment and a smile in my community.
- I cheer for other women. I genuinely celebrate their success and let them know how happy I am for them.
- I ask for help so I don't feel alone and as though I am drained. When I have good energy, I am turned on rather than switched on.
- I schedule holidays before I get tired and need a holiday. Burnout prevention is a priority.
- I move my body with lots of variety. Doing one thing only doesn't fire me up.

- I gravitate towards more books, less screens and have creative and social outlets to channel all the feels.
- I enjoy my work so much it isn't really work. It's more a piece of my life that brings me joy and helping women boosts my libido.
- I believe that my life is incomparable to any other woman's, so I keep my eyes on my own lane and keep following what feels good for me.
- I know when I am getting close to cracking and need rest. And then rest.
- I avoid over-committing as it usually means I end up in martyr mode. Flowing with all the moving pieces is important to me.
- I put a love note in my online calendar for when I have to pay bills because it's an honour to be able to pay for what I use and what makes life enjoyable.

When I meet a woman, I can already feel her libido because it's in the public realm. From the moment we shake hands or gently embrace with a peck on the cheek (or not at all), I'm privy to her libido. Almost instantaneously, I'm given exclusive access to her orgasmic capacity, wealth (not always monetary), appetite, power and her comfort with the edges through her eye contact, wit and laughter.

Even though your libido is out there, you can still keep your sexuality private. If necessary, keep it covert. It isn't for everybody to know but it is for you to find out.

She keeps it in the now

Being a sexual woman is about describing your libido in the

present moment – not drudging everything up from the past as evidence why you aren't sexual or enough. The sexual woman knows that all we have is the present moment.

In this very instance, your libido is whatever you want it to be.

Rather than describing your libido as *flat, non-existent, crappy* or *missing*, could you try bringing it into the now? Instead of tilting towards the negative, could you describe your libido as *curious, wanting, eager to learn, listening, absorbing* and *non-judgmental*?

Every word you choose to describe your sexuality and your libido shapes its form. If there is something to be gained from keeping it flattened and deflated, you already know the words to use. But, if you hold a thread of hope that your libido has the potential to be fully realised and expressed, use words that encourage that. Your libido is listening.

Her libido isn't linear

In a snapshot of life, it's easy to see how many variables can get in the way of your libido – illness, pregnancy, moving, festive seasons, grief, menstruation, burnout, work demands, boozing, the postpartum period, conflict, shame, stress and isolation. It's inevitably going to waver and the sexual woman trusts that when she gives it space, it will come back.

When I delved into exploring my own sexuality in 2012, I assumed it would have a clear trajectory of taking me higher and higher with each, and every, new learning. Not only that, I presumed that experiencing certain types of pleasure once meant that I could re-access and re-create them at my will.

Mmm it doesn't really work that way.

Later that year, when a wise woman gave me permission to not chase my sexual experiences, I was instantly relieved of the burden to be my own maestra. Striving within my sexuality was like slamming down a big rulebook to an intangible entity that seriously doesn't care for rules. From that day on I learnt that my sexuality doesn't respond to rules but it does respond to guidelines. It likes little nudges of *this is possible – wanna try?* over *this can and will be done.*

If I could draw a picture of my libido, it would look like Mr Messy from the children's *Mr* book series. One big, pink, squiggle. My good girl may have coaxed me to do more than a few things by the rulebook but my libido is the least linear facet of my life. It's an unruly force that won't be told what to do or when. In fact, its rebellious and changeable nature makes me love it that little bit harder.

She has an astute inner critic

The sensitivity of our libido doesn't alter with the progression of time. Tellingly, more time in the online world does not give us a more steely resolve. Your astute inner critic is the one that pulls at your sleeve or gives you a kick in the guts when something doesn't feel right. You don't have to be subjecting yourself to explicitly sexual content to see hypersexualised portrayals of women that possibly make you feel inferior.

When you feel that tug on your elbow, that's your cue to tweak your inner world to be on alert and recognise hypersexuality in the media for what it is – a surplus of one very bland ingredient. When you catch yourself noticing that you're being sold something through a sexual filter, can you ask yourself if that's what you would want your sexuality to look like, even if you had the choice? Is that image an accurate reflection of what your libido looks like on the inside? I ask this because I don't believe an authentic libido needs to be overt and gratuitous.

An authentic libido doesn't exist to arouse and serve another person. It exists to serve you.

Your libido wants you to be critical about what you see and hear so the real stuff can come through. Being critical doesn't make you bitter or negative. Your astute inner critic will make you clear and your libido will thrive because it loves clarity.

Regardless of what it looks like on the outside or how your erotic power shows up, you are a sexual woman.

FOUR

Permission to feel safe

I USED TO THINK THAT SAFETY WAS BORING. Truthfully, to me, safety meant a lack of risk taking, a deficit of edginess and stagnancy with life and choices. Look closer and it's easy to see how I saw safety as being equal with the not enough or scarcity mentality.

Now, I recognise safety as the ultimate permission granter to sexually opening. Safety is essential.

Your safety will secure your pleasure.

Safety has since come to mean something else entirely to me now that I've had very visceral experiences of what it is to live without it as my guiding light.

Frankly, I've gone into the edgy endeavours of sexuality work with my 'yes' and my 'no' all over the place. In my hunger to learn all the most sensational, headline worthy aspects of Taoism, Tantra and shamanic practices, I allowed my sense of safety to be overridden. Safety became the last priority because I saw it as the party-pooper of sexual exploration and I wanted to keep clocking up experiences and upping the ante. Writing this now I feel that familiar flush of shame and while I want to give you specific examples, I know that these learnings are just for me. Much like the last chapter says: *your sexuality is personal*...likewise – my sexuality is personal.

What I can tell you is that because of this steep learning curve, my radar for bullshit and creepiness now runs at high voltage. Emphasis on the *now* part. That radar developed its accuracy over time from the things I've done where there was a little reluctance, a good dose of *yes* and a sprinkle of *this could be weird*. A few things I regret, most I wouldn't change for a thing.

Your radar might already be on a wavelength that knows your answer is a flat out *no* straight away. Mine is clearer with that flat out *no* now that I'm really listening to it.

If you're still fine-tuning your own radar for your 'yes' and your 'no' – know that you're getting there. Feel a sense of safety that you're working towards getting your head and heart around your very personalised signal system that exists to protect you. When safety within your learning and expansion is prioritised, you get to where you want to be a lot faster, with a lot less to undo later on.

Taking this to a very physiological level, you and your nervous system are hardwired to feel safe. Studies have proven that our sexual network doesn't turn on to its full potential unless the security centres in our brain are switched off (unless feeling scared turns you on, which is rare).

Have you ever noticed how you struggle to open up sexually to an intimate partner unless you feel safe and comfortable with them and the space that you're in?

Sure, your body might still be able to physiologically open to intercourse and penetration but if your heart is closed, you probably don't fully feel pleasure and comfort.

This isn't helped when we are taken further from safety within ourselves by opening our bodies when they just don't feel like it.

When safety isn't prioritised, your body will find a way to send you the message – *I speak, but you don't listen.* Some common ways your body might say this is by turning up the volume on your pain, creating disharmony within your menstrual cycle and increasing the tension on your pelvic floor. All of this leaves you in a position that makes sexual contact a challenge.

It does this for your protection and only when it can't get through to you any other way.

Safety is the foundation from which you transform your sexual tapestry. It's a struggle to make personal changes in the face of fear, and pushing through or striving can be potentially harmful. These are response styles that are applied to gym workouts and competitive reality TV shows – not ways of nurturing your very tender libido. Translating these hard and fast approaches from the gym to your bedroom can be damaging and may work to hold you back.

Wade into the waters of change slowly rather than dive deep quickly to embrace each shift.

I believe that the potency of any good quality sex education and inquiry can be sourced from its bottom-up approach (as opposed to the top-down approach). What this means is that you're moving with your body's hierarchy of needs through the traditional chakra system instead of going straight to the upper echelons of intuition and transcendence.

Safety, tribe and home come first in the root chakra; sexuality, sensuality and creativity come second in the sacral chakra. Although no one chakra is superior to the other, you're better positioned to reach the higher states when you first tend to your baseline needs of safety and then move into sexuality.

Getting comfortable with safety allows for a little magic to spread throughout the rest of your life. When you feel safe to be sexual, you're fortified to carry that strength with you into every other situation: public speaking, self-promotion, giving from a place of love, receiving praise and above all, feeling worthy of going for what you want.

When I say this, I think of my client Evelyn. Her status quo in life was to take all of the attention off herself as much as possible. Early in her process, she recounted how she would very reluctantly attend her work award ceremonies. She would only ever wear black to them and would stall to get up and accept her awards. Once she was up there, she would run off the stage as soon as possible and go on to hide her accolades in drawers so no one could see. Although she came to see me to feel open to a new relationship after 20 years of being independent, it felt like how she treated her awards, and being acknowledged in general, played a bigger part of her intimate and dating life than she realised.

Her daily life was being reflected in her sex life.

So when she sat before me for her last session, there was absolute glee on her face. Not only had she successfully moved through her ongoing avoidance of pap smears, feeling no discomfort (one of her intentions for seeing me), but she relayed a situation that previously would have caused her to hide or go completely silent.

By learning how to feel safe within herself and own how what she has to contribute in this life is important, she noticed that she suddenly felt comfortable being surrounded by men – a *lot* of men. She took this one step further by giving her personality permission to shine through witty banter and laughter rather than staying silent and getting the job at hand done. When we finished sessions, she hadn't found her partner yet but she had certainly found herself.

You can still have a sexual revolution whilst playing it safe

Revolutions are slow. The ones that create long-lasting change are those that keep the focus on the unfolding part. Your sexual revolution might look like a gentle variation of the following: you start by reading a book about sexuality, then you do an online course, then go deeper with 1.1 sessions and later move into expanding and connecting on a retreat. All might collate to create your revolution. Not all of these steps are necessary though – maybe this book alone will do it.

With each and every offering available to you, ask yourself if it's a *yes* for you. You're under no duress to learn when there's a *no* (in fact, you won't learn much in this state because safety has given way to fear). The emphasis is on gradually collecting pieces one at a time so that you'll be wading into the waters, not feeling like someone is holding your head under the water.

When I've tried to ingest too much information at once,

rather than emerge from my investments upgraded and renewed, I've emerged frazzled and confused.

Frazzled and confused happens when my nervous system has received too much sensory input from too many sources. Whether it was too much personal growth work in the form of workshops, books, retreats and courses; all I know is that I didn't prioritise my safety because that growth was being driven by a fear that I could never ingest enough and if I can never ingest enough, I can never be enough.

Fast forward a few years and I now know that more information will not necessarily make you clearer (I think the *hoorah* from my nervous system was audible!). Most importantly, and this step is often neglected in favour for speed, whatever you learn, your body needs time to integrate. Safety needs the space that integration provides.

Integration is a place of respite so that you can determine what you want to keep of the experience and what you want to let go of. Allowing integration to take up space in your learning is as simple as staying for the corpse pose for the last five minutes of yoga class, taking two extra days off after a retreat or workshop to reflect rather than going straight back to work and staying in the bed with your lover for 10 minutes when sex has come to a close.

Trouble shooting when feeling unsafe

Permission opens the floodgates on opportunity but as you may recall, it doesn't mean that the opportunity has to happen. That's where your consent kicks in. When moments of fear envelope you, permission might need a lighter hand. Before even considering the opportunities and options, scale it back to:

I give myself permission to give myself permission

Anxiety and negative anticipation love nothing more than wallowing in the obstacles that are blocking your true power. The simple words above are a powerful rebuttal to break free from feeling like you are being driven by forces out of your control.

Rather than being in false surrender to fear, also known as tolerating, allow ownership to become the director of your next move. Strangely enough, when we declare that fear owns us in that moment, it starts to lose its power and we begin to own *it*. The next step is to shift the focus on to safety.

I give myself permission to feel safe

Fear will find it harder to exist in the face of external and internal safety. Align these forces as best you can to ground down and let your root chakra know that you are prioritising it.

Planting your feet on the earth or your bed is a concrete action of grounding. When you feel safe here, take it further with placing a hand on your heart and one over your pussy or womb space with your legs open as far as your body will allow. My key words of coming into safety are holding and grounding. I say:

I've got myself
I hold myself
I've got me

Because you do, and you will.

Sexual safety within yourself

Women talk to me about how much they love their partner and the oodles of non-sexual intimacy that flows between them. That part is well nurtured, but their sex life is a struggle that they avoid. Naturally, she's coming to me because she can't work out why they have this conundrum. She'll say, "if I feel so safe with them, why doesn't it feel safe to be sexual with them?"

They are living in safety but there's a gap they can't see. Her safety within herself is the gap.

This is the crux of permission. If the bases of safety are covered from every angle and she still doesn't feel safe to open then it is likely that she doesn't feel safe to open to herself. The next step is to change the chain reaction to become:

I trust myself and I trust my vulnerability
so I can now open up in safety.

Generating safety within yourself has some simple antidotes. Before implementing these antidotes, anticipate some very normal avoidance and resistance as sourcing safety calls for us to go inward for the solution. True safety lies inside of you and this can be confronting. The alternative is that safety within yourself will be ever elusive and external input will continue to fall short in meeting your safety needs.

Could you step into safety by owning your identity as it is now? Not your perceived identity as it will be once you achieve all these other things such as; after you get married, hit a financial goal, have a baby or reach a certain career pinnacle…but right now?

Safety for me needs evidence to anchor me down. My sexuality needs concrete proof that it can be safe and feel safe. In those untethered times, the proof needs to go beyond journaling and mantras. My body needs to meet itself. More work, effort and input with my partner couldn't touch this one in the early stages of my sexual awakening. Stepping to the side to go inward on my own both bolstered my safety and solidified my sense of ownership.

The antidote to feeling unsafe within our self is self-pleasure in all of its forms.

Safety through self-pleasure

The term *self-pleasure* has multiple meanings.

When it comes to discussions about sex, I define self-pleasure as the act of masturbation, but masturbation just feels so heavy. Self-pleasure is lighter. In a broader sense, self-pleasure is embodied through acts that touch on joy, trust and your sense of stability, that also provide comfort and acknowledgment. Think of self-pleasure as an opportunity for pure energy input when you are so accustomed to energy output to others, to your work and to achievement for the sake of achievement.

This is what happened when Emily began to self-pleasure after the dissolution of her long-term relationship. Now in her 40's, she started self-pleasuring for the first time and it quickly turned into her new version of dessert (her words). It wasn't that Emily didn't feel all the usual feelings that go with learning to self-pleasure like boredom, wanting to put all her vulnerability back in a vault, and craving external validation rather than doing it herself, but she chose to keep her focus on the feelings of safety and self-care that it provided her with.

Safety and the freedom to feel safe on her own with her sexual energy was the key to filling a void that she often sought out through her sexual partners. It also equipped her with the resolve to establish her preferences, trust her instinct first and set boundaries that started with her sourcing where her 'no' was. Self-pleasure was a powerful entry point for Emily getting clear on what true sexual empowerment feels like when her only prior understanding of it was that *sexual empowerment and orgasm belongs to men.*

Good quality self-pleasure is structure-less and without an agenda. Whilst it shines alongside time frames and parameters, it doesn't assign itself to a chronological list that needs to be ticked off.

When you hear the call to prioritise self-pleasure, it's helpful that you approach it from all angles in a variety of contexts. You need to know you're safe when you touch on self-pleasure through the acts of:

- sitting at a café alone
- reading alone
- bathing alone
- exercising alone
- shopping alone
- travelling alone
- going to a workshop alone
- receiving a wellbeing treatment alone

Gather these as evidence of safety and you increase your chances of feeling safe about being sexual alone.

Before having babies, I went on a self-pleasure holiday alone. At the time, I was pretty burnt out from nursing and I needed to recharge my batteries and reset my internal compass – solo. It was an exercise of trust, safety and ownership. I trusted myself with my destination (far north Queensland), my accommodation choice (spot on), what I packed (enough to sustain me) and how I spent my time (a perfect balance of energy output and energy input). With my trusted sexy resource of *Urban Tantra* by Barbara Carellas, I was decidedly taking my sexual energy to a new level too. This holiday wasn't a reason to avoid – I saw it was an opportunity to up-skill and a new, luscious environment would be the perfect backdrop for installation and integration.

I recall a pivotal moment where I was leaving Nudey Beach, and I felt this sense of unfolding that was about to happen. I just knew the temperature was my favourite – 27 degrees and pitch perfect humidity. As I walked through the rainforest back to my room, my body was juicy. It was humming. My need to play with this magic through self-pleasure was urgent. The time, the space, the down-regulation had all opened me up to being alive with pleasure. On that popular trail from the beach to the hotel at 5pm, I glanced around and gave my pleasure relief with touch. I felt safe to go there with myself – nature beckoned.

And now my body has this memory. A memory of trust.

Feeling safe to go there with yourself is the ultimate act of trust.

Repetitive trust feeds safety.

When you play with your sexuality in private, you get used to how you move, sound and act when you're in the moment. On a heartfelt level, you're not just feeling yourself but you are seeing yourself. If you can touch on a sense of comfort, seeing yourself in your sexual nature, then it's more likely that you will feel safe within yourself for sex with your trusted partner.

One way to do this is to connect with what it actually looks like when you're in the midst of pleasure, rather than assuming what you look like. Daunting as it may be, a mirror can be one of the most useful reflections to confirm how real you are when you're in pleasure. Before I was a sexologist, a sex coach set this as a homework exercise and I quickly got why.

I saw myself, not just in orgasm but as a whole woman in pleasure. The judgment dropped. The acceptance flooded in. I owned how I looked in orgasm and committed it to memory. From that moment, being natural and sexual was synonymous and less of a big deal.

When I got that evidence, it felt like my own version of normal. When I owned my normal, I was better prepared to go there with Ed. Self-pleasure became a solid training ground for dropping the self-judgment, tasting vulnerability and being sovereign in my ability to give only to myself. Refreshingly, it's also one of the sacred acts of this world that doesn't encourage a selfie or a social media post to mark the occasion.

Self-pleasure isn't as scary or as daunting as it sounds when you have a framework for it. But me simply saying: *now go and self-pleasure!* probably isn't going to light you up and could potentially cause you to feel more resistance. If you need some guidelines to get started, I have a gentle self-pleasure practice at the end of this chapter.

A few words about getting into self-pleasure and taking action with the intention of advancing your learning…

I recommend attempting self-pleasure twice within a two-week time frame rather than committing to self-pleasure challenges (such as self-pleasuring for up to 30 days straight) unless you're already comfortable with it. The downside of completing challenges is that you risk putting pressure on being sexual by draining your libido rather than stimulating it.

When I did a 7 day pleasure challenge as a part of my sexological bodywork course in 2014, I could feel my shoulders slump a little by day 6 and 7 because I *had* to go into my special room and self-pleasure. The curiosity started to drain away as the pressure to do it arose.

Realistically, you can learn just as much by one self-pleasure session each week over a year rather than enforcing a daily self-pleasure practice that you end up dropping out of due to exhaustion and indifference. Slow and steady builds the pleasure.

The world feels a lot less scary when you've gone to the edges of your personal sexual exploration. This is one of the bravest and most vulnerable journeys you can take.

It's safe for you to feel safe.

Deep breath.

SELF-PLEASURE GUIDELINES

Mantras: *I am safe to explore my pleasure alone.*
I am safe to be sexual alone.

Firstly, create a new space in a different room of your home and make it welcoming and warm. Use your creativity with scents, lighting and colours.

Set your intention: There are no expectations here. Something along the lines of *I am getting in touch with myself* or *I am making space for my erotic energy*. Set the timer for 25 minutes.

Breath option: sacral chakra breath – 2 quick inhalations through the nose and one long exhalation through the mouth – try and add a low pitch sound to the exhalation in order to use your voice like 'oooohhhh' or 'ahhhhh'. It's OK if it's a mouse squeak; some sound is preferable to no sound.

Using a mirror, notice your pussy. Explore all of her curves and depths and come to see how everything is positioned. If you are going well with this, send your pussy some love and appreciation as a source of gentle strength and femininity. Think about your history with your pussy and where you have been together. Take 5 minutes for this step if you can.

Once you have done this, begin your self-pleasure and exploration. You can stand, kneel, sit or lie – whatever works. Just try and stay upright so you don't get too tired or go straight into habitual stimulation. Use different types of pressure and touch – kneed your skin, gently pinch it, use circular motions, tickle and tease. Coconut oil is great to explore your body sensually and you can bring in different materials with different textures in to drag over your skin.

Regularly use belly breaths and sacral breaths to re-connect with your body and close your eyes to visualise the blood and energy flowing to your pussy and throughout your body.

There is no pressure to orgasm or have high levels of arousal, this is about re-building the foundation of your sexuality.

Enjoy yourself and incorporate mindfulness – let thoughts flow in and out and pause if you need to. Use your intuition when moving your body – dance, stretch, move.

When the timer has gone off, ground. This is where you place both hands over your pussy to contain the sexual energy you have just generated. Take a moment to say 'thank me' if you can. Then take 5 minutes to lie in the stillness of corpse pose and integrate. Be kind to yourself. This time is a sound investment in getting in touch with your sexual self and sense of safety.

FIVE

Permission to shelve desire

"What do I want?
I want to want to have sex."

ELEANOR GIGGLED. I SMIRKED. It certainly wasn't the first time I've heard this. The want for the wanting is a common complaint of women that feel stuck in a sexual rut.

I get it. I really do. Pre-sexology studies, I wanted to experience the desire part of sex and intimacy so badly. I seriously thought I could will my relationship to just stay in the early phase of the wanting forever. When it inevitably waned, I wanted that feeling back and I didn't want to have to go through a series of steps to get there. It's the ultimate paradox. I wanted the thing that I didn't have but it's trickier than a straightforward exchange of me getting what I ask for. Really, wanting desire for sex and my partner was like hungering for hunger when I felt full.

When my clients echo one of the earliest conundrums in my own long-term relationship, I feel as though I could spend hours talking about it but she wants the short version and she wants it to work now. It's in these moments that I question why I wanted to take on one of the biggest challenges on Earth –

helping women to feel a libido they don't think they have. A lot of actually helping women comes back to helping her re-jig her connection to and understanding of desire.

I had a warped relationship with desire when I thought it would just land in my lap. What I was reluctant to accept was that I had to go looking for it and take action to invite it in. Desire makes life beautiful, and sex scenes in films unforgettable, but the very real fact is that both you and I as a species, can continue to survive without it. This is a little sobering and somewhat unsexy.

Unsexiness aside, all this means is that we need to have our survival comforts taken care of *before* we can call in desire for our sex life. Our survival comforts are feeling loved, acknowledged, safe and respected in our intimate relationships. Sure we can have sex without these components but the problem is for the most part, we don't *feel* like sex without them.

It makes me think of all the times I had sex to try and gain approval and that special feeling of belonging with the other person. These memories strike me with a sudden hit of pain. This particular flavour of desire for sex often (read: *always*) came with a lot of pain. The sex was hot and firey but once it was over I was instantly met with this feeling of rejection and abandonment. Several months of allowing my love and desire play out in this way meant that I started to associate having sex with being something that hurt me.

If this resonates, you might be wondering why even though the rejection and abandonment parts are missing, you still aren't feeling it for your now-comfy, long-term relationship. Could it be that you aren't feeling desire to belong in your union together because you already know (and have proof) that you belong? When you feel satiated and full in these ways, there isn't a lot of need to chase sex with purpose.

Eleanor began to understand. I told her how normal all of this is for women. But we can't leave any of this on the note of 'it's normal so there's nothing I can do about it'. That would be a waste of curiosity. It's from this point that we can start looking at what she can do and how she can become her own game changer to nurture her relationship in all of its parts.

The fruitless venture

Throughout my years of hearing and listening, I've learnt that women want to touch on desire, speak desires language AND fully feel it in every part of their being. We want the full strength version, none of this half-baked stuff. Yet, if we chase desire, and are looking for it in the dark, we usually end up more lost and frustrated, especially when it comes to how vulnerable we are in sex. Wanting to feel sexual desire and interest when we just don't is a bit of a fruitless venture that can cause frustration to climb and arousal to plummet.

To move on from this, you need to step back from desire – it's too full on. Too charged.

Instead, I suggest you start with information. Curiosity. Understanding your basic feelings. Quietening fear. Taming disgust. Releasing shame.

Clearing out in the form of a purge allows you to create space before you invite something new in. Putting desire and wanting on top of pain, active trauma and suffering will trigger more *I'm not enough* and *I'm less than* when it doesn't work.

So let's shelve desire for now.

While we're at it, let's drop goals and expectations too.

All of them create pressure that you really don't need when you're giving yourself permission to be sexual. You might have noticed that this book isn't littered with goals, exercises or boxes to tick. I've done this purposefully to move you out of that achievement mode when it comes to sex. Sexual ownership needs to be on your terms and carried out in your own, unique way.

Shelve desire and befriend incentive

What few people outside of the sex geek community know is that studies have confirmed humans to be incentive driven when it comes to our magnetic attraction to having sex. Motivation and incentive boil everything down to the question: *what's in it for me?* When we're so used to looking outward to nurture others as givers and caretakers, this question can create serious discomfort. After all, isn't it selfish to think about sex in this way?

Well, no. Remember that the sexual woman isn't selfish but she is self-centred. There naturally has to be something in it for her when it comes to her going for what she wants in life and sex.

Have you ever had sex when it feels like there's nothing in it for you? No acknowledgment, no attention, no care and a whole bunch of fumbling around so that your partner can get off? This universal experience creates the opposite of an incentive to return to sex. Rather than getting juiced up, you're probably going to feel de-motivated and deterred from seeking it out again.

Sex isn't a selfless act and when I've treated it that way, I've come to feel pretty bitter and resentful about it because I wasn't allowing myself to be 50% of the interaction. Incentive works for me when I can't yet feel desire because it propels me into this very primal action mode. It's less a case of *what is already inside of me that wants expression*; more *this is what I can go and claim because I am driven to.* Incentive works especially well when there are glowing memories to draw upon because I have evidence.

If you don't have evidence in the form of positive experiences or memories of sex yet then your incentive to have sex will be to create one (or more).

Asking yourself, *what's in it for me?* allows you to source your own pull towards your partner. For many, orgasm on its own creates incentive but even if you are orgasmic, you probably require another angle because sex is more layered than just releasing tension. Perhaps there's an incentive to feel a hard to come by feeling like bliss; to receive a unique sensation like shuddering with pleasure or to be in a position of power that feels taboo.

Putting yourself first in this way symbolises ownership. If you can't feel an incentive that is solely for you then bring it into the context of your relationship.

Can you be incentivised by sex that cements your reunion after you've had time apart?

What about sex that shows you both still have the ability to be cheeky, playful and nothing like the way you are in the monotony of daily life?

Neither of these possibilities require desire to take the lead. But they do draw upon the ingredients mentioned earlier like information, curiosity and understanding.

Desire will follow incentive when it has space to insert itself and that space comes when you re-balance the experiences of intimacy in your relationship. I've noticed that this intimacy imbalance usually plays out in the form of women saying to me *we spend so much time together and do everything together but we don't have a sex life.*

Desire and incentive struggle to find a place in the midst of enmeshment, which is when your identity and needs are so closely intertwined with your partners that you lose yourself. Be on the lookout for other forms of warmth and intimacy that are actually strangling your sexual intimacy. Healthy space from your partner and having individual identities are necessary if you want to feel desire.

Adopt the Mr Messy model

Permission to shelve desire means swapping the mathematical graph of continual relationship improvement for a much more erratic model. Instead of one straight ascending line over time when it comes to sex and desire, I propose treating your relationship just like I approach my libido. Yes, Mr Messy is back in all of his big squiggle glory – messy, unstructured and unpredictable. Can you tell I'm a child of the 80's?

When Marie came in for a top-up session two years after we first worked together, there were a few mindsets we needed to iron out around desire. Together for 15 years with her only sexual partner, she said: "everything has been really good since I last came in for sessions but recently, sex has sort of stagnated. You know how sex should just keep getting better as time goes on? Well, that isn't happening and I want to get the desire back".

The attachment to our relationship constantly and consistently progressing and improving is bound to cause us frustration when we hit roadblocks.

Before our discussion could progress any further and I could really start to help Marie, I needed to normalise that there are no *shoulds* in a committed relationship, and that sex doesn't place itself on a linear graph of advancement. Sex and our libido are going to respond to all of the U-turns, disruption, grief, trauma and upheaval that await us all. When we take the pressure and emphasis off the line graph concept of sex and desire, we can exhale and move into a state of trust that what is now isn't forever.

So, what can we do? I suggest that in order to touch on desire and a subsequently better sex life, we first need to begin to love sex. If it feels impossible to love it then we need to at least like it. Or not hate it. Attempts to guzzle pleasure on top of variations of dislike are futile, discouraging and at worst, stunt your sexual journey. This is what I propose…

You have to like sex before you love it

Traditionally, desire has strong associations with love. If you want to love your sex life and you just don't right now, this is your prompt to scale everything back to basics. The leap from dislike (and even disgust) will be too big and daunting. In keeping with my approach to wade into the waters, you need to like sex before you love it. As positive and affirming as the word love is, it might be too strong for where you are. Make *like* your new bar to meet when it comes to sex.

By shelving desire and inviting incentive in, you are essentially keeping the focus on what you like about sex so that you'll be incentivised to have another taste. If you draw a complete blank when it comes to what you like about sex, that's OK. There's more to clear and more to come. Your boundaries will be the best informant of your desire because they will tell you what you like, don't like, what needs to stay and what needs to go. We'll get to your boundaries in the *Permission to have boundaries* chapter.

After I scrunched up the line graph of continual sexual improvement with Marie, we got down to the question: *what does she like about sex?* Like so many women, she didn't know. This is the point where it's tempting for women to ask me: *can you tell me what I should be liking/desiring/loving?* Only Marie can answer this question.

Acknowledging our preferences is a key part of forging ownership and empowerment.

A bonus to dropping the hunt for desire is the permission to drop the expectations and high-end fantasies that perpetuate avoidance. Unless you are actually going to create that ultimate fantasy scenario and space to have mind-blowing, transcendental sex then it's time to come back down to Earth and claim your sex life for what it actually is, not what it could be in an alternate reality.

Prue came to this realisation when she said: "The sex that we have isn't going to be moody and hot, passionate…where everything is new – we aren't going to have that. Instead we're going to have a real world connection". In that moment she gave herself permission to shelve desire, because the yearning for it was actually inhibiting her taking that crucial first step to getting intimate with her partner. Before self-sourcing permission entered, she kept doing the same things and waiting for desire to magically step in. Essentially, she moved from passive wanting to active ownership.

When we stop pining for the far-fetched fantasy that we have little incentive to create, we can start to enjoy being in the comfort of our present relationship and sex life.

It's empowering to know that our own version of incentive will take us back to sex that feels good and this incentive might just make space for desire to come out and play (but no pressure).

SIX

Permission to trust

THE MOST EXHILARATING (OR SCARY) PART of permission is that it changes you from you requiring an external source of input to an internal one. Granting your own permission essentially re-wires you to ask yourself first, before you ask someone else what the answer is. This shift is the key indicator that you are being controlled less by your good girl and owning more of your emerging sexual woman. Your sexual woman is alluring because she knows that:

More ownership and trust =
less dependency and validation.

Being in your good girl mode is limited. When the good girl dominates, there is no end to the loop of asking yourself:

'did I do this right?'
'did I please everyone else?'
'did I do this good enough?'

Flip it around and being a sexual woman feels infinite. When your sexual woman is holding court, she asks:

> 'did I please me?'
> 'was this action true for me at this point in time?'
> 'was I guided by my feelings rather than rules?'

As we saw with the golden trifecta, permission doesn't stand-alone. One of its closest sidekicks is with trust.

Trust is one of the activating components of permission.

When I notice that highly functioning women have a block to trusting themselves, I am quick to ask: *what evidence do you have that you shouldn't trust yourself?* This question stopped Elise in her tracks.

At 31 years old, Elise was seeking help in opening up to penetration when her body had never allowed it. With a steady analytical job, safe home and very supportive husband, everything in Elise's life was just as she orchestrated it and she couldn't think of one step out of turn that gave her the impression that she couldn't trust herself. Yet when it came to asking her how she felt, she would always have this pained look of doubt. If her response didn't start with the words *I think,* then she would say *I feel...*(look at me with an eyebrow raised) and then say her feeling in a way that was slow, questioning and ultimately seeking my stamp of approval. She trusted her mind implicitly but she didn't trust the feelings within her body.

We dug deeper. I asked her what aspects of her life she could trust to anchor this feeling into her body. She paused and said she could feel trust and presence in her weekly basketball game. In basketball, she trusted the process of relying on other team members and them on her, that she needed to act and be responsive to support the objectives of the game and that above all, she doesn't want to get hit by the ball (which never happened to her). It was an analogy I could use to prepare her for what is in store as she navigates her feelings in life and sex.

Her trust in her ability to play basketball all came back to a skillset she has repeated, the confidence that she can respond because of that skillset and that above all, knowing that she is a valued contributor to the team. A lot like sex really.

If vivid memories of an episode, or chapter, in your life arise which feel like proof that you can't trust yourself, then take a moment to weigh that brief space in time up against everything else in your life where you've taken a chance, or listened to your instinct and gotten it right.

Those moments when you nailed it.

Those instances when you followed through and felt good feelings.

Even if you did have a chapter in your life or a number of experiences that weren't in alignment with your trust, ask yourself, *what did I learn from that time? How did it take me to the next point that truly did work in my favour?*

When we give ourselves permission to trust, we remove ourselves from the limitations of dependency.

Permission is a green light –
trusting, inward, affirming.

Dependency is an amber light –
pleasing, external, validating.

The words that you use when you're in permission mode will be so different to those that you use in dependency mode. Just to prepare you, your language and mindset will probably be different when you step forward and fully own all your stuff and that includes your sexuality. You'll begin to feel and sound like you.

Trust that it will come back

When I'm in the midst of one of my own emotional shit-storms, I'll be honest…

I don't trust.

The loop in my fear-based brain is so predictable and even more convincing. It gets hooked on the *always* – that everything as it stands now is a constant. Permanent.

I know it's hard. I know right now feels equal to forever. But your juice, mojo, passion, zeal, libido and sexual fire *will* come back. It will come back when you invite it, encourage it, learn about it and move with it.

I say this for you. I say this for me.
When it all feels so far from you…
Trust that it will come back.

Not trusting, despite evidence to the contrary, is a default of mine. The longest episode I ever experienced of distrust was when I was pregnant with my second daughter. My falling pregnant with her was a complete surprise (yes, sexologists can have surprise pregnancies!). At the time, I felt like my "big plan" for 2016 was going to be BIG. I was well into the swing of my business and feeling like I was doing my best work. I was so amped up to go deeper into my offering of bodywork and public workshops that I could feel the buzz of arousal swirling in my body.

It wasn't so much the positive pregnancy test that put all of that to a halt but the way my body was responding to the pregnancy. I was nauseated and lethargic beyond the first trimester. My spirit was dulled. I didn't glow like a pregnant woman is supposed to. My ideas and quick wit were reduced to naught.

Creativity is sexual energy and I just didn't have it.

Throughout my pregnancy I didn't have sex or self-pleasure. The only time I did self-pleasure was to get the baby out after a 40 week gestation. Honestly, the acupuncture was more effective than the forced orgasm.

During the entire 9 months I didn't trust.

I wanted to fold my business.

I never wanted to taste pleasure again. What was the point? I couldn't feel it anyway. Wine had no spark and coffee had no zing. Going out into the world felt like a tease – a stroking of my exposed bones through the gash. Being out there felt like everything I *didn't* feel was thrust in my face.

I felt like a sexual fraud. No, it went deeper than that. I was certain I was a sexual fraud.

I wasn't embodied.

I resided in lack.

And I was really fucking angry about it.

The disempowerment of an already challenging pregnancy was brought to fever pitch when I received a diagnosis of a basal cell carcinoma (BCC) on my face when I was 16 weeks along. A BCC in itself is not necessarily that big of a deal but a BCC that plants its roots and leaves rogue cells close to your eye and brain when you are chocked up full of human growth hormones is a potentially big deal. It was an ordeal. Cue fumbling, misogynistic doctors, too many appointments, lots of time in waiting rooms and two facial surgeries in one week with an active 32-week foetus. I didn't feel anything close to hot or turned on. I felt disempowered and frozen.

In this time of disconnection from my wisdom as a woman and a sexologist, I watched lots of cooking shows. And I napped. I was convinced that this would be my life: working for the man, cooking shows and laying low. Anyone looking in right now can see that this is a temporary state. People would say to me – but you are growing a human! My response was, *yeah, I know. But I want to grow a human AND do what I normally do.*

At some points in this protracted state of distrust, I had enough insight to ask myself, *what am I learning from this?* I came back to this question as a habit that was instilled during my time learning sexological bodywork. This somatic approach to people's sexual blocks taught me so much about presence, sensation and trust. Above all, trust. No one can tell you what you are feeling or why. But we can always ask – *what did you learn?*

As I asked myself this question in 2016, I drew a blank. Then I'd usually cry.

The learning is that sometimes we don't know what we are supposed to learn from challenge, pain and struggle until we are through it. Such was my case.

I needed to be patient and wait until I was out of the early postpartum days when I was still livid about how deflated and powerless I felt for the year. Little pieces were revealed to me month to month but it wasn't until I had completely moved out of the hormonal upheaval and back to having a menstrual cycle that I could see exactly what I needed to see. Before then, it was all too close because I was *IN* it. One of the key learnings of 2016 was how I'm presented with the opportunity to surrender and how I push against it.

Instead of napping in surrender, I napped begrudgingly.

Instead of pausing work in surrender, I kept pushing.

Instead of recuperating in surrender with cooking shows, I lay there feeling guilty.

Sound familiar?

Not your usual surrender

The themes of my story are familiar terrain for so many women. We want to surrender so much but we want to stay in control because we don't trust. Surrender is the fodder of romance novels – the heroine is ravished and swept up by the hero as she allows him to exercise his power over her. You can feel the erotic charge of not having to do, or be, anything but to follow the lead of someone magnetic…someone who knows what they are doing. Someone you trust.

I didn't get surrender for a long time and I've come to recognise that it isn't just me that missed this learning. Somewhere along the way, lots of us confused tolerating for surrender. When women say 'OK' to sex they really don't want to have, they aren't surrendering to their partners; they're actually tolerating. Persistently tolerating leads to resentment and bitterness and that makes it really hard when we are saying that we are keen to feel interested in sex.

To get a picture of surrender, we need only look back to the heroine in the romance novels. She has the right idea. She's empowered through her ability to surrender. She isn't passive or weak and she certainly isn't tolerating. She's an active participant in the process and she's driven by a willingness to be open not by controlling the situation but by flowing with it. She's immersing herself in the ingredients of non-judgment and curiosity. Above all, she trusts herself and trusts her hero.

When we surrender, we are saying yes to the other person touching us for their pleasure. We too get pleasure because there's nothing we need to do – something (hopefully) wonderful is being done to us. This is the paradoxical medicine that so many good girls need to feel the things they really want to feel.

I better own that one…this is the paradoxical medicine my good girl needed to feel the things she really wanted to feel.

Shifting over more of your life to surrender can be a hard slog. Minimising it down to the words 'just surrender' isn't going to work – trust me, I've tried that one many times! Playing with surrender in your daily life and sex starts with the small stuff. You need a comforting doorway to usher you through to this expansive arena.

What surrender means to me

I admittedly fumbled around with this notion of surrender for a long time – not really connecting to it. Through a long and windy route, I found the easiest way to connect with surrender wasn't through using the word *surrender*. It was the word *allowing* that permitted surrender's true colours to shine bright for me.

When I allow something in my life, it means that I trust that I'm exactly where I'm meant to be. Yes, I cry about it. Yes, I feel a sense of injustice over things not materialising how I want them to. What allowing ultimately means in my life though, is less pushing. Less pumping stuff out and forcing creativity and specific, tangible outcomes.

When I get on one of my good girl binges, my output becomes ego fuelled and (surprise, surprise) people pick up on that. What I've taught myself to do instead is feel my intentions, put my invitations out there, and turn up when there is a yes. I try to always keep the flavour of putting myself out there without attachment. I come home to the belief: *I trust myself and I can hold myself.* It isn't anyone else's role to hold me unless I specifically ask for it and they want to hold me.

My version of surrender also means allowing the aspects of my personality that are an enduring part of me. This grants me permission to factor who I am into all of my decision making processes. I'm always going to be a high achiever who weirdly forgets how long it's been since I last washed my crop top. I'm always going to have a fast burning body that needs to eat 6 times a day. I'm always going to be a helper who goes the extra mile and thrives off connections with other women.

Allowing in life makes for allowing in sex.

Moving into a space of allowing in sex

The very idea of surrender in sex might be causing you to curl up into a tight ball. You can't even imagine "go with the flow" sex, in fact the idea of it spells serious anxiety – how can you go with the flow AND control the outcome? Let's scale it back a little. Try the word *allowing* and see how that feels to you instead. Allowing kind of takes the power back because you can ask yourself: *what will I allow to happen in sex? What will I allow to happen to me in sex?*

Your partner can't take from you in sex if your consent hasn't allowed it. There's a classic kitchen scene that has irked millions of women for millions of millennia and it shows what happens when we don't allow.

You're standing at the kitchen sink daydreaming, cleaning and organising but checking out into another world. Your partner walks up behind you and grabs your ass and proceeds to go into a bear hug from behind. You immediately go on guard. You might stay quiet for a moment and tolerate this touch you didn't invite in. When it gets to boiling point, you shake them off. It's not that you don't want affection, it's that you don't want it in this version.

What the fuck just happened?

Nothing throws a woman off more than touch that she perceives to be sexual in a non-sexual situation. Sure you might want to be adored and shown displays of affection but what happened in that kitchen felt sexual to you, not affectionate. You were being taken from, but not in a way that you had you in a state of allowing. Rather than the hero and the heroine scenario, it was the hunter and the hunted. You didn't want to be devoured, you wanted to be adored. Those lines are extremely thin.

True allowing means that you can let the cards fall for a while. Wouldn't that be a relief from being switched on all the time?

Surrender and allowing in your sex life is a clear display of trust.

If you want more surrender and allowing in your intimate life then play with it using the edges of touch. Surrendering still has some parameters guiding it. You can make requests for types of touch, on parts of your body, for specified time frames, that let you experiment with a feeling of allowing. These parameters need to be conveyed and honoured for trust and surrender to grow.

Imagining surrender is a safe way to test the waters before trying anything new in real life. The following may give you a gauge on how you can soften into surrender. They are posed as questions rather than must-do's. Always remember that surrender and allowing need your consent.

Can you allow your partner to squeeze you tighter and longer than you usually prefer when they greet you?

Can you allow your partner to kiss you the way that they want for 2 minutes?

Can you allow your partner to give you a non-sexual massage on a part of your body that you specified for 5 minutes?

When there is something tangible to try and work with, we start to build trust by gathering evidence, solid evidence. Yup, it requires doing something new but remember you've conquered so many new things in your life that felt daunting at first.

The most potent advice about trust that has stayed with me came from my clinical supervisor when I was working as a nurse. At the time, I was in the thick of burnout, which is exceptionally common for nurses who work with clients experiencing drug dependency. My whole nervous system was set to the fight or flight responses because my body kept receiving the message that it was an unsafe environment to be in.

Yvonne Lumsden, a fellow ex-nurse and now Kundalini Dance teacher and Reiki Master said something pivotal to me. She said:

"Rather than sitting across from a client and saying *I don't trust them, I don't trust them* could you instead say to yourself: *I trust me?*"

And that was it.

I was taken aback. Holy shit, how did I not ever think to turn it around and shine the light on my own empowerment? My own sovereignty?

I trust me.

A seed was planted that day to allow my internal permission granter to emerge from right down deep. She was just buried under a whole heap of fear, rules, regulations and stipulations that didn't ever inform me that first and foremost I could trust myself.

Not long after this, I went on to complete my sexology studies and wade through the waters of personal growth. Even though I lapsed from the truth, *I trust me* at times, it never left my soul.

Now I beckon you forward to say the same.

I trust that it is there and
I trust that it will come back because
I trust me

SEVEN

Permission to be choosy

BEING CHOOSY IS THE SAME AS BEING FUSSY, RIGHT? That word instantly suggests that you're high maintenance and somehow snobby.

Well, you're not.

You're refined, selective and yes, choosy. Own it.

I'm not here to convince you that you should like something that you just don't right now. I've learnt the hard way that solving your sex problems isn't a matter of persuasion.

What I *am* here to convince you of is, your own quirky blueprint as a woman and how gentle acceptance of what is will accelerate your learnings far beyond what someone else thinks you *should* be.

Learning about your own sexuality needs to be a process of honouring your ability to choose what you *do* want. The ability to give yourself permission to go there and question what you want will bring to light the acts within sex that are a 'yes' for you.

At the heart of it, being choosy is about using your consent, and that's a good thing. Your body will know the difference between an external source stating *this is how you need to be more open* versus approaching your sexuality with the questioning mindset of *where can I try to let more of what I want in?*

Choosing your sexual partners

When you recall your history of sexual partners, it may be necessary to breathe deep to gently give yourself some compassion about the times when you weren't being selective and choosy. You did what you did at the time for whatever reason that felt so compelling, whether that was pure arousal and desire or a medley of intoxication and seeking approval. Try not to let any shame or regret overshadow all the choices you're empowered to make today. Your intuition wasn't what it is now. Twist it around to think of how you have been equipped with a laser focus within your intuition because of those transgressions.

As of this very moment in time, every person you allow near, close to or inside your body will be chosen by you.

Sometimes in sessions, I work with women who need to feel more at peace about not choosing more sexual partners. She sits before me, now in her late 20's, 30's and beyond, explaining to me that she's only ever had the one sexual partner. At some point in her formative years, she made a conscious decision to only share her heart and her libido in the form of sex with one person and one person only. Whilst she usually has no regrets about who she chose, she's left with this questioning of what else she could have felt in the arms of another and if it's her lack of "experience" that has her feeling blocked and stuck.

Julia was a woman who I would describe as choosy. She was also very comfortable with control. When she came to see me, she explained that she only had the one long-term sexual partner. She was neat, and had her shit together in an analytical job, yet felt very disconnected from her libido and potential to enjoy sex with the man she loved. She was quirky and endearing when she turned her nose up as we discussed the female anatomy.

When we dug a little deeper into why she felt inhibited about sex, she confessed she had a fear that if she opened up to her sexuality, she would become addicted to sex, like a switch that would go from zero to overdrive. I assured her that learning more about her sexuality at 31, and remaining choosy meant that this was very unlikely to happen.

What Julia was really saying to me was that she feared losing control of herself and her ability to be selective. She was intensely worried that her wild woman would step in and dominate her without her giving her the green light to do so.

During our time together, we kept the focus on staying choosy with the assurance that she could be more open to sex when her nervous system was in a gentle state of down-regulation, instead of stress and disgust. She needed to know that she could be herself even when armed with new knowledge about her body, breath work and sexual positions. Julia's anxiety about becoming addicted when she was avoidant worked as a timely reminder that our head can leap into far-fetched fears that we will act like an entirely different person in sex.

The reality is that we can be ourselves in our choosiness and be sexual. There doesn't have to be a conflict.

Choosing to be sexual

When you're in the dark and your libido feels like it's just suspended in limbo, without direction, it's empowering to come back to the truth that being sexual is a choice – a choice you can choose again and again. The ultimate lesson here is to be choosy and make choices. Just don't be so choosy that you eliminate all the options and all the choices (and hence, take no action).

Permission to be choosy entails being a bit of a sexual rebel, but not a rebel in the traditional sense.

It's seeing the latest Cosmo article on all the faddiest of sex tips, and not falling for the hype.

It's about noticing something that tantalises the masses when you can see clearly through the veneer.

It's about moving from giving a shoulder shrug and saying *I like everything* and instead saying *I like this and I don't like that.*

In your choosiness you choose not to succumb and emulate the "ideal" woman.

Sometimes being choosy will feel like you're the only one that hasn't drunk the sexy Kool-Aid. Resist the urge to follow the pack if it doesn't feel right. I've witnessed women who knew that they had a preference (i.e. were choosy) have their consent breached by being coerced into doing what the rest of the group was doing. Actions like these rob our sense of empowerment and cloud our consent.

Have I followed the pack blindly before? Yes – all under the guise of giving myself permission to *go there*. Little did I realise that my being wild and liberated could have done with a hefty dose of being choosy to keep my actions aligned with my heart. At the time, it wasn't clear whether I was going *there* for me or going *there* to stroke the teacher's ego.

When you're tempted to stray, stay close to the fact that being choosy is empowering, and that feeling safe within your own decision making process makes for a very sexual woman.

How to be choosier if you aren't already

Women's personal stories are littered with themes of not being choosy with life options because she didn't feel good enough to go for what, and who, she really wanted. At the heart of it, it's more than she doesn't feel deserving, it's that she doesn't feel *worthy* and outsiders love to look in with quick judgment and say: *she settled.*

Possibly. But we don't really know the full extent of her backstory – maybe a big part of the problem is that she grew up learning to take the first thing that comes along or she would miss out completely. Perhaps she got used to being comfortable with someone (or anyone) rather than no one at all.

Not being choosy might spell a carefree, go with the flow, life for some women but if you're feeling like who comes into your life and your body time and again isn't aligned with you, then becoming choosy could give you the gift of personal health.

After working with hundreds of women that are worried about what other people think of them, it's easy to see why we are fearful of being choosy and it's because we don't want to be seen as fussy or too much. Think of a time when there was something that you really wanted to buy or own and you settled for something less or your second choice.

Did you walk away completely at peace about owning your second choice?

Or did you walk away with that niggling dissatisfaction?

I think of that dissatisfaction as the longing that can't be quelled.

When we settle for second best again and again, we're living with the mindset mantra "that will do". Maybe trauma has convinced you that you shouldn't go for what you want. Maybe someone didn't treat you respectfully and left a mark that bruised your dreams and your worth.

Whatever the origin, does it feel possible to gradually move away from "that will do"?

Not being choosy shows up in life and sex as:

...taking the first offer that comes your way rather than assessing the options

...spending time with anyone that will spend time with you, even if it doesn't feel right because you believe being with someone is better than being alone

...living constantly with a this will do/they will do approach to your possessions, jobs, homes, friends, income and partners

...making sure that someone else is happy regardless of how uncomfortable it makes you

...always feeling like being choosy, particular, or having standards in life and sex is OK for other people but not for you

Becoming choosy requires exploration into your feelings of self-worth. The more solid your self-worth is in the now, the more likely your choices today will go on to influence and create the life and future that you really want.

Choosy is the circuit breaker of low self-worth.

If a part of your not being choosy involves lots of decision-making on the fly, rather than you taking your time, trust that becoming choosy will mean valuing patience and moving slowly over being impulsive. The *Permission to take your time* chapter will allow you to go deeper with this reflection.

The least threatening way to edge your life forward into worthiness, is by making a declaration to prioritise your worth and change one small thing. I've found the safest way to do this is to choose an aspect of your life that bothers you, something that you really value that you don't prioritise, that could be really easily corrected. It could be as small as buying the brand of tea that you really like at the supermarket, over what's on sale or the cheapest.

Getting comfortable with the everyday ordinariness of the supermarket can get us used to questioning the value of our bigger life choices, like our partners and careers. The small things can reflect the big things.

Such was the case with Abby. She has a massive heart and her needs would often get lost in her relationships with men who needed looking after in some way. Now in a relationship with a man who loves her more than she loves him, she started to acknowledge that it wasn't so much that all her partners shared a common thread of mental health diagnoses, but that she was always staying with them because she was waiting for them to reach their potential. In a weird twist, she too wasn't living to her potential, only none of them were putting it that way to her.

At 30 years of age, she was now tired. She went so far as to say: "My judgment knows it isn't reassuring that one day my needs will get met." Self-worth that is paralysed with doubt is often holding out for the *one day*.

Rather than look specifically to her relationship in that moment, we looked at her "playing small", as she put it, and rubbed a big highlighter all over her potential that wasn't being reached, and the ways her intuition was screaming to be heard. She undoubtedly had the heart, wisdom and disposition to start her own energy healing business (and had even registered the name) but kept stalling because of the lucrative aspects of the job she was in. That niggle to change was getting louder though and she was struggling to work out of alignment for much longer. She didn't want to "leave her heart at the door anymore".

For Abby, it was about stepping into two new, big, beliefs: firstly, that she was worthy of taking her time with her entrepreneurial dreams and secondly, that it was safe for her to live in alignment. She and I both knew that without these two anchors, very little would change in her intimate and work life. Interestingly enough, as she did this, her love and desire for her partner grew, making her more willing to tweak the aspects of their sexual life that needed attention.

If your intimate life feels overwhelming right now, it might help to develop a sense of mastery and confidence around that non-sexual step, just like Abby did with her business idea. Alignment, sovereignty and ownership in the non-sexual realm will make you better prepared to take action when it comes to your next sexual step forward.

When it comes to moving into healthy self-worth, over time, you will naturally flip the script from:

It's not safe for me to be with someone good for me

TO

It's safe for me to be with someone good for me

Because being choosier means feeling more alignment and more enjoyment.

Being more particular means that you feel more presence because you feel safe.

Sometimes women feel solid with their self-worth by day but they become clouded when intimacy is the key driver.

When Georgie had decided to date after still feeling raw about a breakup with a man that couldn't meet her needs, she observed how she feels intimate with other men very quickly. She admitted to me that she was distracted by the variety of men out there but her ego really liked it.

Throughout one particular session, we spoke about a man Georgie was seeing, but hadn't had sex with. She had set a date to catch up with him, but wasn't really sure what the driving force for spending time with him was. She was confused but wanted to keep the date because she had set it up. I put to her that she could cancel meeting up with him but, in that moment, Georgie didn't feel that it was safe for her to change her mind. She was too concerned with how it would affect him and his feelings.

As our discussion deepened, Georgie came to a realisation. She said: "my nurturer inside wants to look after him. I have a pattern of wanting to fix and nurture men. I've always been in the caretaker role. I'm using my sexuality and men who are needy find it attractive."

We used the rest of our time that day to explore what Georgie's heart wants and to prioritise this over what she thinks she should do. I left her with the question of, *what would your dream relationship look like? What would your dream relationship feel like?*

Regardless of what has happened in your sexual history, or who you have been intimate with, you are worthy of being sexual with people who make you feel good.

You don't need to say yes today just because you've always said yes.

You can say no to having sex with someone and trust that this will give you the confidence to allow a more ideal person to come in.

You are worthy of taking your time in sex, you are worthy of garnering attention in sex, and you are worthy of enjoying sex.

When we don't feel worthy, we often don't feel safe to even dream or consider what we might want and what the best possible version of that is. But something that feels far away from us doesn't mean that it's far-fetched.

To become choosier, could you make a little space to dream right now, even when what you want feels far away?

I've been both in the spaces of not being choosy and being choosy. More specifically in my own story, I was really choosy about my sexuality to the point of repression, then I expanded past the threshold of choosy into a kind of shamelessness. I bounced back shortly after into safe contraction and being choosy in the healthiest way. In my strange version of coming full circle, I now see choosy as synonymous with maturity.

Becoming choosy allows us to have the life and sex life we are worthy of.

That's the power of choosy.

How to be less choosy when it paralyses you

Softening your need for everything to be a particular way can be a little terrifying. Let's make it easier by breaking it down into what parts of your life are non-negotiable. When you know your non-negotiables, you can see what is presenting itself as a must, but is really a cover story for procrastination, avoidance or even sabotage.

Your reflection into the paralysis of choosy also calls for some reasons versus excuses exploration. One thing I've noticed about women experiencing blocks with their libido, is that the reasons and excuses not to have sex have persisted for so long that they have intertwined, condensed and been repackaged as one and the same.

The default to being choosy has developed a very pointy, fixed end. Yet, when women separate their reasons and excuses not to be intimate with their partners, they're repositioned to be empowered and to choose a more constructive, and restorative, way of saying yes and no.

When we know an excuse is popping up, it's an opportunity to diffuse and clear the air. But excuses posed as reasons render you choice-less. They stumble out of your mouth as fact. Your excuses hold so many answers. Strangely, your excuses are where growth lives because excuses give you valuable insight into the needs you are denying yourself.

Think to a time when intimacy starts heating up and you feel your partner's arousal building. Out of habit, you feel the excuse arise and break it all off. This happens within seconds. Go back, look at your excuse and comb over it like a valuable piece of data.

Saying that you have something else of pressing importance to attend to, like the housework or an email, can be interpreted as a kind of sabotage but also makes the statement: *I need to be present to experience intimacy with you... I need to be more focused than I am right now.*

Notice the difference between the feeling of, *I want to avoid this altogether,* and the feeling that, *this isn't the right time or space.*

That is the power of excuses versus reasons.

Your reasons will empower you to propose an alternative, like a different room in the house or to get sex started in 10 minutes when you're less distracted. An excuse on the other hand will put a stop sign to sexual intimacy for as long as it can weasel out of it.

Look for the clues when your tendency to be choosy is getting too rigid. Use your choosy to course correct and soften. Use it to receive instead of give, even with the smallest of acts. Use it to inform you as to what time of day will work better for sex, when morning feels too jarring and 10:30 p.m. feels too late. Find your optimal windows of time and space and be sure to distinguish your reasons and excuses.

Reasons honour you in that moment whilst excuses keep your sexuality at bay.

Being choosy is a pathway to acceptance

Being choosy is liberating when it gives you the chance to drop comparisons with other people and come to a place of acceptance for how you've been perfectly and uniquely designed. Allowing all of the external noise to fall away, so that you can remain focused on your lifestyle, is a sure way of feeling much more satisfied and at peace with what plays out in the bedroom.

When Nina came in for her final session with me, it was astounding to hear what had shifted for her when it came to accepting the reality that she always has and possibly always will experience physical discomfort with sex. She made a choice to reframe her very personal and unique sex life with her husband instead of allowing her mind to go into comparing what she thought it should be. She said, "I accept that our sex life is different to what I see in the movies. I have confirmation that my relationship and sex life isn't mainstream. My whole thinking about it has changed. If I really wanted to have sex, I can because the potential is there. We just have a different way of starting off in the bedroom (due to her experience of pain and discomfort). I'm accepting that my situation is a slower process than others but sex is still possible".

It's never too late to pivot and own your choosy as Carol came to accept in sessions. It took her a while to understand that her ability to choose enabled her empowerment. Now a kind-hearted woman in her 50's, Carol had enjoyed the benefits of swinging with her husband for years. To be clear, Carol was selective about who she shared her body with in the swinging community, much to many other swingers dismay.

She recognised that when she made a choice to say *no* when it wasn't a *yes*, she owned her power. She said: "I like the freedom and the choice of swinging. The peace for me comes from saying I'm OK with my choices within the swinging community and I'm OK with my choice to swing in a world that doesn't understand and judges swinging".

Carol being choosy allowed her to access her safety, and therefore her pleasure and liberation. She carved out her own place in the world, which gave her the superpower of knowing that she's OK, regardless of what anyone else thinks.

Especially through my work with clients, I've learnt that being particular, choosy and maintaining standards are traits to standby. So, I will encourage you as I encourage them when it comes to staying choosy about:

...who you share your body with
...what type of touch you like
...what your sexual space looks like
...what you choose to influence your libido
...your contraception
...your sexual toys and aids
...your energy expenditure
...your intention for sex
...how you define intimacy with your partner
...what matters to your identity

When women give themselves permission to be choosy, they are armouring their bodies, hearts and souls for the best possible reasons.

It's this armour that will make your libido for life and sex chink-proof.

That sounds kind of badass, doesn't it?

EIGHT

Permission to love vanilla

BEING SEXUAL ISN'T A TEST.

When I treated it like a test, I ended up striving and being goal orientated. In my experience, goals, pressure and my precious female libido are not good bedfellows.

When I first wrote online about being a sexologist that was in love with vanilla sex, it was like I could exhale. There was nothing I needed to try and reach for anymore. I finally began to own that all of my learnings had melted and melded together to become their own version of *Lauren.* Arrival is a sweet, sweet place for your libido to land. Permission will move you closer to this.

When it comes to sex, vanilla is my favourite flavour.

Coming full circle after trying nearly all the flavours – Tantra, orgasmic meditation, sexual healing sessions, embodiment retreats, Taoism and I even certified as a sexological bodyworker; to emerge the other side loving the original flavour felt like an act of defiance. Looking at the ice cream smorgasbord of sex, I chose the plainest flavour over the rainbow one. (Who does that?)

When you start learning about sex there can be a tendency to go all out.

To bare all, to release and uncover.

To burrow right down a rabbit hole of self-exploration.

It's never demanded of us that we take this approach, but curiosity usually wins when it comes to the hunger to know and live as deeply as possible. Activating our sexuality after waking up from a long slumber has such allure. The word *addictive* comes to mind.

That's where Tantra comes in. Before I completely woke up to my real world life (and Tantra loves to herald that you aren't awake until you meet it) I finally owned that Tantra and its subsidiaries had cornered me into pressure and expectation. As a youngling, Tantra inspired me. I had bug-eyes. Now emerging as a wise woman, I recognised that all I felt was not enough because there was some elusive pinnacle that I needed to strive towards.

Cue light bulb moment.

If I don't want to be striving and trying to achieve in my sex life, I definitely don't want other women to either. Chasing the elusive is out of alignment with my ethos. More importantly…

Pressure is the antithesis to female sexuality.

It all started to slot into place how I didn't fit – anywhere really. I had to truly feel all the resistance to learning how to switch my trusty clitoral orgasms for deep vaginal ones. Or revelatory cervical ones. Or enticing nipple ones. Or full body ones. I glanced at the books with a look of dismay and thought: *I just couldn't be bothered.*

A number of years ago I read an article that debunked the categorisation of female orgasms and went on to call any orgasm 'the female orgasm'. In that piece, permission was granted for those of us that help women to remove the experience of orgasm from some kind of system that women need to progress through. Despite this permission granting moment in the literature, I can say with certainty that the old *clitoral orgasms are inferior* mentality is well and truly thriving in the Tantric community and this disgruntles me.

Didn't we abandon that highly damaging and oppressive belief system last century?

Isn't the message of sexuality work all about coming together and connecting as we are, rather than fuelling disconnection and segregation?

Permission is about coming as you are and being empowered to stay as you are.

The biggest inconsistency about Tantra is that it's advertised as a come as you are approach but so much of the undercurrent is about striving higher, fully transforming and unlocking a code. And to get the code, you need to be part of a club. Individuality gets lost in a place like that.

My burning question to all the women out there is:

What if what you are doing right now already feels really good?

What if investing your time into changing your pleasure pathways results in feeding the not good enough mentality?

A mentality that millions of women already feed all day long.

When I realised that I felt irritated about Tantra, I decided to move on and get real with myself. The word *authentic* had lost its authenticity and real was the only way that it was going to be for me.

Real is that I'm a mama of 2 with a 7-seater wagon in the 'burbs that was not having hours of Tantric sex and multiple orgasms. When I looked back and questioned how big a discrepancy there was between some of what I endorsed in my practice as a sexologist and all the shortcuts I took in my own sex life, I felt the familiar flush of shame.

I wasn't living Tantra because it wasn't real to me.

If Tantra isn't tangible to me, then it's not tangible to the women that I am here to serve. There's a problem there and my next phase of service called for me to rectify that.

Being able to grant yourself permission means being fully informed. There is so much beauty in Tantra when it's practiced with integrity so, before you step into any space that claims to enhance your feelings about your sexuality, please familiarise yourself with these Tantra pitfalls.

The (mis)use of the word energy

The best thing I ever learnt was to try and avoid using that word. *Energy* is too big, unclear and vague. When you are describing a personal experience in your body and you can't use the word energy, everything changes. Notice when you can't resort to the word energy how you have to become crystal clear on what it is you are experiencing, feeling and sensing. Being precise about what is happening to you and within you is what will get you closer to the power you crave. If you can't find anything else that fits then use energy, just try to use it sparingly.

Complex processes to reach transcendental experiences

I can tell you now that the instructions to have a full body orgasm are not easy to follow. Neither are most of the Taoist ones in *Multi-Orgasmic Woman*. Reading pages of a recipe and trying to go inwards simultaneously is really not sexy. More to the point, I don't think good sex needs to be complicated, long winded or take years to master.

Here's what I propose: what if you simply tried to learn one new skill a week rather than a whole lot of skills at once? Go for easy and steady learning over complicated and intense – you'll see progress and feel more encouraged that way.

The multiple definitions of Tantra, the myriad interpretations of it and the spectrum of practitioners

Tantra is a big umbrella. How can we discern what and who is honourable and has integrity and what and who doesn't?

The best advice Danielle LaPorte gave at her Brisbane event was 'if they feel creepy, they are creepy'. Danielle, where were these words for me when I was starting out?

You may hear the words 'integrity', 'alignment' and 'consent' leave people's mouths but the truth will speak in volumes through their actions. And on the note of speaking volumes, watch out for the loudest voice confusing you into thinking that they are the most convincing and thus, the most truthful. Just because someone is loud, doesn't mean they are honourable.

Naturally, the sexuality community talks and I'm at an advantage of being connected with some high integrity members that keep me informed of the quality of other practitioners work and what their real message is – I mean the one they spruik out of the public eye. Once curious about some of the offerings out there, I would say that now 99% of them trigger off a *no* in my body. Unfortunately, violations of participants consent and safety are commonplace, and this danger stems from the practitioners desire to becoming widely known as being edgy, breaking new ground and pushing the taboo.

All of that is dangerous because it's taking place to feed their ego, not your learning experience.

What training practitioners have been through is also another big question. Are dangerous practices becoming systemic because most people are doing the same training and walking away thinking that boundary violations are normal?

Simply by being in a shared space with some Tantra teachers, I have felt some serious unease arise in my body. I can only articulate it as there is darkness overshadowing them yet they work in the field of proposed enlightenment.

In any personal growth circles, the word *boundaries* will come up, as it does later in *Permission.* Knowing your lines in the sand in each moment in time is what leads us to our own personal state of health. Yet within Tantric circles, it isn't uncommon for practitioners to have thousands of Facebook friends, not followers on a business page but friends, because it allows people who do follow them to feel like they are getting exclusive access to all of the practitioner's most inner thoughts and perspectives. This is a matter of personal choice but it works like a really sneaky business move – allow people to feel like they know you, like reaaaally know you so that they start chanting the doctrine of you and sharing your work because...you're *friends* after all.

When it comes to navigating the blurry lines of social media, I made a different choice. I have personal pages and business pages. When women work with me, we both need clear lines about how they are the centre of the process. It also gives me the choice of what I want to share with a client and to ensure it's relevant to what she is learning and exploring through sessions.

Am I going to invite every person online into my inner most world of home and family life?

Well, no. Because...boundaries.

Language that is elitist

Language is powerful. Tantric circles that use words and language that are big, all encompassing, and vague are elitist. When words are used to create separation rather than its purported connection, we encounter some serious exclusion and triggering.

A one or two week Tantra training doesn't mean that you are entitled to use terminology that has little or no relevance to your culture or heritage. And there will be some terms that are steeped in a deep ancient culture that people think we have a right to use because hey, it *sounds* profound and enlightened.

Perhaps we have come to believe that the more someone speaks in riddles, the wiser someone is and the more we need to internalise their message and outlook on life.

Sharing from the place of *I* is really powerful and humanises a message, but if you find yourself reading a whole essay from a Tantric practitioner filled with the word *I*, know that the essay isn't for you. It's a dear diary that has been made public so that you can crave to be insightful like them. Stirring the pot of envy and creating this desire for you to emulate them is a big drawcard to get you to become dependent on their work.

For far too long I played along with a nod when I heard certain terms that don't have any meaning unless they are expanded upon. Beware that when you step into some Tantric spaces, you will encounter terms like *holding space, feel your energy, embodiment, transmutation, call in more Shakti/Shiva* and references to goddesses and archetypes that you may have never heard of before. None of this you have to subscribe to if it feels alienated from you. If you don't understand, do not nod and stay quiet like I used to. Seek clarification by saying: *I don't understand, what do you mean?* Simple language is effective language and we should all understand the concepts being conveyed and how they apply to our real world life.

Coercion under the guise of learning and expanding

I'll admit that I've said *yes* way too many times under the guise of learning more and going deeper into Tantra, spirituality and embodiment. I deliberately ignored the feelings of *that's not right* in order to learn more about my identity and my sexuality. Essentially, I pushed change to happen beyond my level of readiness.

Was I coerced at times? Yes.

Coercion happens when people tell you to use your intuition, but are all the while manipulating and withholding information from you to generate a desired outcome. Hint: it is for their gratification, not your 'self-discovery'.

Over the years, my naivety and hunger to learn had me disregarding what my gut was saying. I've been in spaces where the consent of participants was not sought. I've been in spaces where people were pushed to express way beyond their comfort zone. When this happens, people feel unsafe and unprocessed trauma can re-emerge. On a really personal note, because of my adoration for some of my former role models, I feel a sense of shame for all the times where I may have pushed a client further than they were ready to in the name of exploration. If this is you, I am sorry.

Even after I wrote my first article on vanilla being my favourite flavour, I had Tantra practitioners contact me trying to coerce me into advertising their events. I say coerce because they weren't actually asking me, they were telling me what was going to happen. Long after I said no the first time, they continued to ask in various different ways and added further insult by suggesting that I would benefit from attending their event. I believe that how other practitioners communicate with me is a reflection of how they communicate with their clients and the expectation I sensed was: *I will get what I want and I know I am right.* When I'm asked to just advertise something for someone who I don't actually know, I can feel the entitlement seep through the correspondence and it feels completely off.

Again, if they feel creepy, they are creepy.

Simplification of women's deep concerns and trauma

I've tried not to eye roll when I hear classic Tantra exercises conveniently inserted as an answer to women's questions about their feelings towards their partner. There are so many catch phrases that are almost put on repeat that it becomes nauseating. Phrases like: *how is that working for you? Do you want a breakthrough? Whose voice is it that is saying that?*, consistently fail to address women's underlying issues. It shouldn't have surprised me when a healing session with my medium revealed that she had already seen a dangerous Tantric practitioner I knew at work and could recite his catchphrases word for word years later. It was haunting to say the least.

These are the real concerns of women that continue to be overlooked in Tantric circles:

...feeling pressured to have sex when they don't want to

...feeling that they need to be someone they aren't in the bedroom

...knowing how they can switch into feeling like sex amidst everything that is going on in their daily lives

...learning clear communication skills that work

...sourcing the permission and desire to have sex and initiate sex

So if you get the call to dive in, here is what you need to know before you access Tantra:

Choose someone that you trust

Follow practitioners of the Tantric community closely for as long as you can and if possible, try to get honest opinions from people who have already accessed their work. You will know by the way someone speaks about their experience whether they felt empowered and opened up through their participation, or whether they left feeling uneasy.

If your gut intuition says yes, attending a workshop or online learning is a great way to get a feel for their approach, what they stand for and to ascertain how comfortable you are learning from them. When choosing to take that learning privately, safety, trust and rapport will be the most important ingredients in working one on one with a therapist, coach or teacher. Most importantly, know that when you are in a learning space or group, you never have to do anything you don't want to. Take what information you want and leave the rest.

You will need to delve into where your sexuality has been, where it is at and where you would like it to go. Honourable practitioners aren't going to jump in and ask you to aim higher or say that a certain route is the only solution. First, *do no harm* means that they should help you to wade into the waters of discovery and follow your comfort and consent. If you are uncomfortable in sex then you are probably uncomfortable talking about it, so taking that step is a BIG deal. A good quality practitioner will need to simultaneously keep you comfortable whilst you expand.

Lastly, if they offer bodywork, you should never feel pressured to do it and if it's a yes for you, they should always be wearing gloves and clothes.

Learning Priorities

Doing any kind of personal introspection needs to incorporate your life outside of sex. Thoroughly. It might not always be that sexy and you may be in a rush but that part is vital. Letting go in sex is easier if you feel comfortable letting go in non-sexual experiences. Surrendering and being all femme-power in sex is more nourishing and aligned when you feel pleasure with touch, food, fun and laughter. All of these areas of your life need attention and gentle correction before your sexual concerns can be addressed.

Initiation into sexuality work needs to encourage ownership. The surest pathway to ownership is through accurate information about the female anatomy and pairing this with simple communication skills that you can take into your bedroom.

When you can accurately name the parts of your pussy, you are the woman who is confident. When you can say "I would really love it if you could rub my clit" (because clits are AWESOME and are totally the foundation of your sexual pleasure – something that Tantra likes to overlook), you become the woman who is empowered. Understanding and putting a voice to your complete sexual and reproductive anatomy needs to be prioritised in any process otherwise; you will be searching for bright lights in the dark.

If you feel anxious, inhibited and like you just don't get sex, then you may well need to learn how to effectively de-compress. This will be a repetitive process as a part of any quality learning experience because it will accelerate your learning.

Most importantly, if you're in fear or distress, you won't learn.

If you're in fear or distress, you won't open to resuming or starting sexual contact when you are back in your real world life.

You should also be taught how to bring your anxiety down in your body and be taught how to feel more alert if you are overly depressed/asleep in your body (and you want to have sex). De-compressing doesn't have to take long and as great as having a *practice* is (another big buzzword in the spirituality and sexuality communities), if you are anything like me, you will probably view it as another avenue of pressure in your life you don't need. Personally, I would rather just learn a skill in the space of others and then come back to it when sex is getting started.

Yep, you have permission to not have a practice.

Beware going up so high you can't feel the ground

Going down (or up) an esoteric spiral can be illuminating but how much of it are you going to be able to translate to your bedroom? An important step before this is, really examining the basics by incorporating a fresh outlook on your sex life as it is now and making it more satisfying in a realistic way.

I believe that we need to start with looking at what really isn't working and where your *no* is. If your foundations of consent and boundaries are overlooked in favour of higher highs then you'll feel confused when you get home. Even if a session, a workshop or a retreat stirs things up for you to question, it still needs to have a sense of completion by the time you leave or finish. Ideally, you need to be leaving feeling grounded and solid. Beware the Tantra trap of prioritising being high, floaty and transcendental over rooted and stable.

If I had to choose between being grounded and being high, I would choose grounded every time.

When Megan came to see me several years ago to explore vaginal orgasms, I gave her some ideas about how she could delve deeper. At the end of session 2, I just paused. Probing any deeper was going to feel like pushing. Speaking off-the-cuff I said, "you are enough. You don't need to be any more". With her head hanging down and tears streaming down her face she slowly looked up and said "thank you". That was all that her libido needed.

And my best guess is that your libido needs to hear this too.

NINE

Permission to be serious

YOUR SEX LIFE DOES NOT HAVE TO BE FUN AND FRIVOLOUS. No matter how many advertisements you see that project the carefree woman, tossing her hair in her lingerie with a bright smile that says *you aren't this*– you need to know right now that this concept does not need to be your reality. In fact, it probably isn't many women's genuine reality.

Can you own that as a woman you are far more dynamic and complex than simple and straightforward? That this is a better time than any to take that same degree of seriousness that you apply to every aspect of your life and drop it straight into your sex life? After all, your daily life and sex life are one and the same.

You are capable and it's totally possible for you to feel carefree and filled with joy in the bedroom just that…maybe seriousness is the medicine that's missing.

What seriousness has shown my clients and I is that moving towards fun and frivolity in sex and life needs a graduated approach, especially when there is a question of how safe you feel. If letting go and getting playful is on your agenda, try not to skip those in-between steps. There is a gentle order to be followed and it's this:

You need to be serious about your libido before you have fun with it.

At some point, we all want sex to be light and fun, easy and carefree, deep and powerful. The proviso is that in order to get to all that we have to take our libido seriously first.

Your libido is worthy of respect, of being fed, of being acknowledged. When you've done this THEN you can giggle with it, play with it and have fun with it. That's the catch.

Being serious doesn't mean being dull. I now see it more as a means of being bright through being focused and moving with intention. Seriousness suddenly becomes cool when it lets you embrace your knack for being studious and curious. Most importantly, it requires putting a stop to poking fun at yourself as a way of keeping yourself down.

You may have already made jokes about yourself in the bedroom. But we're not talking about a soft laugh to diffuse the tension or reduce the awkwardness. This laughter comes from a place that keeps you feeling like something inside is damaged or irreparable. Perhaps you joke about what kind of a root you are or label yourself something like a "starfish" or a "plank".

When you speak about your sexual functioning or presence in the bedroom in terms like these, it is a knee jerk reaction to your feelings of frustration. More specifically, it's your defence system holding court, working tirelessly to keep your self-worth low. Try as you may to discharge your frustration, when your libido isn't taken seriously, your potential is minimised.

You aren't alone. No doubt you have a lot behind you, as your own inventory of evidence that you shouldn't take your sexuality seriously. It's a classic case of 'what's the point, nothing really changes'. The reason you feel this way isn't your fault.

With so many millions of women having a history (or current reality) of sexual assault and abuse that has caused unquantifiable degrees of trauma, we need to take your relationship to sex and your libido especially seriously. We cannot minimise or joke when it comes to the ways that your body, mind and soul have experienced trauma and breaches of consent.

I've seen many women use laughter to diffuse their deep and persistent pain and Cilla was no different. At 35 years old and married to a man who is devoted to her, she was struggling to safely express her sexual feelings without drugs or alcohol.

Within sessions, she was self-deprecating when she described her sexual functioning and awkwardness. All of that felt like the complete opposite to who the drugs gave her permission to be – the wild woman who takes charge and does the fucking. She was sometimes light about this very long phase of her life that she had now walked away from. She labelled herself all sorts of names and pigeonholed her sexuality to cope with how she felt about her lack of presence during sex, and her persistent sense of not feeling safe.

When I reflected to her that her attempts to lighten the blocks of trauma with humour were keeping her stuck, we began to slowly move into the territory of kindness, honouring and tenderness. She had done not being Cilla in sex and it didn't work. It was time to treat her precious libido with care and to take it seriously.

When you arrive at the place of being ready to move on, you will no doubt realise that you also need to leave behind the notion of it all being out of your control. In this very moment, you can choose to take all of this – your problems and your pain – seriously in order for you to make strides through your blocks and inhibitions.

When we aren't being serious we are leaving everything up to chance.

Rolling the dice on our sex lives, especially when we're in a long-term relationship, can see intimacy go quiet. Sitting down, truly feeling the problems we have, saying *our sex life is shit* and creating a plan doesn't sound very sexy, yet the payoff is that we start to move through our problems with active focus rather than haphazard wishes.

One of my little sex therapy secrets, is that simply starting to pay more attention to your sex life can be the best motivator of libido and arousal. The process of unburdening by talking about it alone can give women the biggest boost in libido simply because she is taking action towards it shifting. Talking is a potent act of releasing and clearing. Maybe the most potent.

When I gave myself permission to name my stuff, I moved swiftly into the zone of ownership, which amplified my libido to become my coolest sexual self. Or perhaps my geekiest sexual self (still cool though).

The language of serious

The way that you speak to yourself will be the biggest indicator of your readiness to move into serious. Rather than not talking about your sex life, or just making off the cuff remarks about it, serious sounds like:

...I'm ready.

...I'll give it a go.

...I respect myself enough to stop poking at my pain points.

...This is fucking hard but I've got me.

Serious might come across as kind of rigid and stuck in its place but I now feel how it has a sense of motion to it. It embraces the opportunity to pause rather than stop and relishes the chance to be in control, which usually demands an action. There's always something at work internally, even when we're at rest. With its careful eye and conscious heart, it's constantly investing and re-tweaking our human experience. Serious knows when we are carefully putting our learning on hold for a valid reason and when we are quitting because it's easier to stay in our non-sexual cocoon.

You may have noticed that being fun and jovial is the tone of sex advice in mass media, namely women's magazines. If you have ever read sex advice that's all about putting the heat back into the bedroom, getting your biggest orgasm yet or doing a sex quiz then you may have already felt that sense of fun evaporate quickly as your very real sexual problems go unacknowledged. This approach to female sexuality isn't fair for you or for me.

I've personally had to do so much unravelling from what I thought sex should be and feel like based on mass media. It was only by stepping away from as much of that as possible that I could begin to choose what my own message of female sexual empowerment was going to sound like. This clear-out of what I no longer needed to hear or subscribe to made way for fun coming in to play. For as long as I tried to put fun and pleasure on top of annoyance, irritation, conflict and distress, I was getting scarily close to shutting down and re-traumatising myself further.

Take serious on holiday with you

Simplistic sex advice can toot a new location as a way of boosting libido and sexual response, but I've found that this approach comes with mixed results. Going on holiday or having a night out at a hotel can put a couple's problem under the magnifying glass rather than absolve them of their sexual issues altogether.

I've worked with women who are left with intense feelings of inadequacy when they haven't been able to have pleasurable, or successful, intercourse on their honeymoon, or to acknowledge another important milestone. Despite how optimistic they were feeling, their problems followed them to the next destination and then back home again.

A new destination is worth a try for calling in more playfulness. Out of the daily grind, women have the space to have more of their parasympathetic nervous system (our relaxed mode) dominating so that we use the phrase *why not?* with a little bit more sincerity and less apprehension.

Holidays used to be so secretly triggering for me. I knew that they were there for connection and I wanted to go on them for that specific reason. Only that, we would get there and I would go into avoidance mode or sabotage mode. It usually wasn't until I got into *really tipsy drunk mode* that sex could happen. Alcohol was always my go-to ice-breaker for intimacy on holidays.

When I decided that taking my life and health seriously would underpin 2018, I purposefully cornered myself into strategising my time off very differently. I couldn't afford the cost that alcohol was taking on my soul and with that out of the picture for our time away together, I crafted my own unique way of getting serious about intimacy so I wouldn't stuff it up.

The first night Ed and I had away from our two girls had an action plan. We only had 24 sweet hours together so we had to use them wisely. On arriving in the idyllic Byron Bay on New South Wales north coast, I had solid ideas as to how we could drop into intimacy quickly – we didn't have the luxury of lots of time or days on end. We went out for coffee as soon as we arrived, to symbolise that we were anchoring in to where we were rather than having our heads stuck in Brisbane. We went to our room and made space for intimacy before we went out to our friends wedding that evening. Making sober sex the priority is in stark contrast to how I used to respond to intimacy when we used to go away. In the past, Ed would initiate sex early on, I'd say no or worse, say yes but come up with an excuse only to say yes later when we had been out for dinner and drinks.

Getting slowly serious over the last 5 years or so has allowed sexual intimacy to be elevated from late and drunk to early and sober. Serious keeps getting me closer to my values, my preferences, my truth and my deepest orgasms to date.

If going on holiday or relocating hasn't brought relief to your problems, know that there is nothing wrong with you. Learning that a change in environment doesn't change what is happening on the inside, is an opportunity to get serious about what really isn't working within your relationship dynamics or your relationship to yourself. Whether at home or on holidays, here are some steps you can take to edge it into new terrain:

- Not joking about your sexual response, body functions or occasions where you feel you lack. I use laughter to diffuse tension and giggle at shared awkwardness rather than to deflate my efforts or keep myself down. Derogatory remarks can come in thick and fast when we don't take our libido seriously. The act of seriousness needs to have a symbiotic relationship with respect.

- Choosing social media and influencers carefully. Your libido is so sensitive to what it consumes. Only follow what enhances your life, not what sucks your precious vitality away or (weirdly) makes you feel like you aren't taking your life seriously enough.

- Knowing the difference between when you are being triggered into feeling not enough and when you are being triggered because there is an aspect of your life that needs love and care.

- Curating your television, film and social media consumption to align with what you want to learn and what grants you permission.

- Addressing issues as they come up rather than sidelining them for a more optimal time. Whatever you do in the present will top some vague notion of future action. Procrastination doesn't play well with serious.

- Getting professional help. A bottled up libido will crack under the strain of not knowing how to get relief. Talking about your sex problems is an act of serious that can't be spoiled by procrastination or apathy. Help may also come in the way of having someone look after your children so that you can go on a serious date with your partner.

When you've gotten serious, you can call in the fun. Here's how…

#1: Get really clear on what fun will feel like in your sex life

From the very beginning, you need to get clear on what your connection to fun is and how that can be translated to your bedroom. Play around and get comfortable with the words: *I'm serious about having fun in my sex life.* When you have sourced the quality or the characteristic you're looking for, you can start to envisage fun or playfulness happening. This is important because my version of fun and your version of fun might look and feel different.

Real fun in sex for me can be summed up with warm smiles, sultry eyebrow raises, using cheesy sexual innuendo, getting sweaty and shared laughter. It can also involve trying one new thing when I feel most open to incorporating a new skill (hint: this is most likely to be in the follicular and ovulatory phases of your menstrual cycle or try a bit of full moon action if you no longer/don't cycle).

Fun can mean giving to Ed in a playful way when I don't feel like receiving.

Fun in sex for me means that we have a laugh, we get really cheeky, we connect with eye contact as we smile, there is a sense of spontaneity and that we embrace all sorts of movement that reminds me that sex doesn't have to be perfectly curated.

Fun sex for you might involve roles, toys, lively music, food, a new location or having a sense of thrill before you have sex like doing something really exciting that brings your heart rate up.

Consider getting serious about the quality first and then get clear on what it actually means to you. Then you can bring that quality into your sex life.

#2: Speak to the fun you created when it happens

When the quality of fun or playfulness that you wanted to bring in actually happens in your sex life, try and speak to it. At the end of sex, if you had sex that was really fun, make eye contact with your partner and say, "that was fun!" (or you can do what I do and drop the exclamation mark to say in a really sultry way with an eyebrow raised "that was fun…")

What those three little words do is create an anchor for that experience. It solidifies and cements fun happening in your sex life and lets you know that you can create new fun memories together.

I know when Ed makes eye contact with me and says, "that was fun!" (even if I suspect he had more fun than I did), just him saying it allows me to look back and see it from his perspective. That kind of positivity is infectious. It's encouraging and it brings more love into my memories of the intimacy we just shared.

The way sex finishes is your prime time to say to each other what was good if there wasn't a lot of sound, acknowledgement or words shared during sex itself. Rather than rushing to clean up, slow down and pay some attention to connecting and closing this special interaction. After sex, or *after play* as I call it, is your chance to communicate the positives and to end on a really feel-good note. Think of it as the taste that's going to be left in your mouth. When something tastes good, you are going to want to come back to it.

#3: Don't become attached to always having fun in sex

I recognise that this is what we're already talking about. Yes you want to call a quality in but try not to set it as a goal or as an expectation for sex. Sometimes this sets you up to feel disappointed and when what you want doesn't materialise, you can be left with more frustration and less incentive to make another attempt.

Really try to go into sex with a very open intention of *I'd like to bring fun into sex.* Saying it in this way is a form of ownership and means that you're not putting pressure on your partner to create the fun in sex. This intention is also keeping the focus on fun being something that you'd like to happen, but it's not an absolute requirement.

Not being attached to it will also mean that when it doesn't happen, the pendulum in your mind doesn't swing to the limitation of *sex is really boring* or *sex is always boring.* It keeps you in a more sensitive mindset that is comfortable with things not always going a certain way. When you feel frustrated, try to be OK with sex just having a sprinkle of fun and not necessarily being full volume fun from start to finish. It sets the bar pretty high for you (and me) and you need room to move and make mistakes.

Sometimes the twist is that the mistakes, awkwardness and squishy sounds make us laugh and it's sweet to realise that it was becoming serious that got us there.

TEN

Permission to stay in control

I'M NOT GOING TO DISCOURAGE CONTROL.

Neither am I going to say you need to surrender.

Because you don't.

It may well be the fodder of romance novels and erotica but you don't need to subscribe to the notions of surrender and ravishment.

Similarly, you don't have to want to be taken by your lover.

Being out of control does not necessarily mean enjoyment and pleasure. If the pursuit of surrender threatens you and puts you on guard, that's a clue that it isn't what you should be aiming for.

In fact, what your sex life may well need is some more control. On your part.

Maybe, just maybe, the medicine you need is to call the shots in the sexual part of your relationship for a little while. I'm talking about moving you from a place of powerlessness, and something being done to you, to being empowered to create the sex life you want on your terms.

This isn't about you disregarding the wants and needs of your partner on a long-term basis. Being in control doesn't need to be permanent. In order to move into safety and comfort, your ability to control when the *yes* and the *no* happen will mark an important phase of re-calibration that edges you towards liberation.

Control will call upon so many of the other lessons in *Permission.* Being in control seeks guidance and support from boundaries, the capacity to speak up, being serious and taking your time.

My question is: when you know control in the other parts of your life so well, why does control feel so incompatible with sex? Inviting control into your sex life might mean that some components of your control repertoire will be tightened and some will be relaxed, and that to me is kind of cool. Yes, you can relax control.

The undercurrent of keeping your shit together

Having your shit together is great in theory but can cause havoc with your feelings. Sure, it paints a pretty picture of how thorough you are, how intelligent you are or how dependable you are.

But while you are getting all your ducks in a row, your body is flaring off signals that it can't keep getting left behind. Being fixated on having your shit together can mean that you treat your life like a machine. You can see where all the pieces fit and it's glaringly obvious when one isn't in its right place. That one little piece can threaten your whole notion of having your shit together.

Problem is, your body isn't a machine and us high achievers usually only realise this when it starts to show dis-ease. The most common complaints I get from my clients are gastrointestinal tract problems, shoulder pain, depression and disrupted menstrual cycles. Your and my need for perfection gets in the way of our bodies natural ability to self-soothe and self-regulate.

On the other end of the spectrum, for those with chronic disorganisation and insecurity, having your shit together is a dose of good medicine to tap into the power of consistency and safety. These are qualities that let us feel alignment when everything feels scatty and haphazard.

Taken too far though, we get tight. Really tight. The obsession of having our shit together causes us to coil up without the spring rebounding to open.

Being sexual requires a releasing.

The very real fact that women have problems with orgasm is synonymous with problem releasing and letting go, but I propose that it's also about being seen. Lots of women can orgasm alone but struggle to completely *go there* in front of someone else.

Struggling to release follows this sequence:

> *I can't let go because if I let go then I will be seen to be a certain way and if I am seen to be a certain way then I will be pigeon-holed this way AND THAT IS A VERY BAD THING.*

It's all worse case scenarios. The limitations of worse case scenarios are that we become cut off from enjoyment and possibility as we continue to succumb to fear and rigidity.

When you start to feel like everything is urgent and that you should have every aspect of your life in perfect order, come back to this list (or even better, make your own). These are the necessities on my own got-my-shit together inventory:

- My home space. Safety is key. Home isn't about what it looks like; it's about what it feels like.

- My finances. Money is empowering and liberating and we need it in more women's hands.

- My hormonal health. This isn't about what I look like, it's about having my hormones in balance, which don't discriminate or determine body shape. Happy hormones for me equals a better libido for sex and life.

- Being as good a parent and partner as I can. Not perfect or necessarily consistent but stable and a safe refuge for my girls and Ed.

The rest can ebb and flow.

Your sexual partners may change – just make sure they treat you with respect and honour your *yes* and *no*.

Employment changes, sometimes a job is just a means to an end. And there will be overlap between study and work and work and self-employment and a lot of that will rarely look clear and cohesive.

Having your shit together doesn't mean isolation

When you've got your shit together, it's easy to confuse being responsive and responsible with the need to go it alone.

That's where we good girls and high achievers have honoured a very misconstrued message. We think that being responsible and having our shit together means being self-reliant. Cue lots of 'I'm FINE!' responses to people's genuine questions about your wellbeing.

Fast forward through thousands of 'I'm FINE!' responses and I can reveal with certainty that the mask eventually drops. The façade eventually crumbles and our truest feelings simmer to boiling point. In this simmering state, nothing feels scarier than vulnerability. In order for our guard to drop, we need to start with trusting ourselves and then opening our arms, hearts and pussies (note: pussy opening is purposefully the last of these gestures) a little wider to trust others.

We can all still be in control and come together. You don't have to choose.

Use control as re-direction, not shutdown

Fi came to see me as a 21-year-old woman who felt withdrawn in her loving relationship of 2 years. Together, we dug deep to uncover some of her blocks that centred around a fear of abandonment if she didn't say yes to sex and an experience of powerlessness when she went through with it.

When I saw Fi again after 6 months in-between sessions, she noticed one significant thing had changed in her sex life to make it feel more positive. She said that her and her partner had tried putting her more in control. I nodded my head vigorously with a sly smile. I asked her why this works well to improve the quality of her sex life. She said: "Me being in control is me knowing that intercourse isn't a requirement/pre-requisite to anything that gets started. But the funny thing is that intercourse usually *does* happen."

I asked Fi why she thinks this trick works.

"It's a work around. The knowledge I'm going to have sex stops it from actually happening. Not feeling obligated means I can enjoy what is happening in the moment without getting caught up in anxiety and stress. I can say *stop*, nothing has to go anywhere and nothing has to happen that I don't want – it's spoken now" (as opposed to being assumed).

What Fi experienced makes sense to me. The paradox of control is that you need to harness it to feel more interested and curious about sex. Knowing that you can wield this sense of control and decision-making boosts your involvement because the pressure is being taken off. The really important part is to use this control in a sort of dance with your partner. Continual shutdown to show a loving partner that you are in pain about sexual issues becomes unproductive. It looks like control on the outside but it actually blocks the course of action. Healthy control is about using that shutdown to re-direct you to safety and an opening, any opening to signify that you're willing to move on.

If your partners want to bring some kind of role, toy or skill into sex and it's a no for you, could you use that no and re-direct it into a yes of some kind? Opening up to that yes gives us the chance to put forward a counter-offer and to keep a dialogue running.

You might not be willing to go into an adult shop but are you willing to browse on a female friendly website to at least have a look?

You might say no to attending a couples workshop but would an online course in the confidentiality of your own home allow for both control and growth to take place?

Healthy control is all about using your anxiety and apprehension as an agent of change rather than trying to play out this alienated role of surrender when it comes to sex.

Really, how natural is it for you to drop into this complete alternate persona as soon as the lights go down?

Yup, it's tough for me too.

I'm multi-faceted but I'm not compartmentalised. If I want to be present in sex, there's no way I'm going to play a different role. That's a spell for me to become disembodied and check-out as I try to keep up with an appearance. Kudos to those who relish it and rock it but when it comes to sex, all I want is to be me.

Being in control isn't dominating

It's easy to get the notions of control and dominating confused but control doesn't mean that you want to be dominating. I've had hour-long conversations with women that centred on her partners desire for her to dominate and take charge. Being in control is different to this.

When a woman feels a sense of pressure to call the shots and dominate (when it isn't a part of her identity that she wants to unleash or even simply explore), she begins to widen the intimacy ravine and move into a state of distress. She will say to me that she doesn't feel confident to dominate but it runs deeper than confidence.

Sometimes, as I sit across from her and propose various gentle entry points into taking charge, it starts to become clear that resistance is her way of saying no when she is struggling to simply use the word *no*. She feels blocked because she, flat out, doesn't want to do it. Other times, it isn't until the end of the hour that I am hearing how much of the request for her to dominate in sex so that her partner can surrender is truly coming from one source – and it isn't her. Requests like these trip couples up because she defaults into believing that becoming something that she isn't in the bedroom is an act of compromise. If she's in a relationship with a man, his frustration about always taking the lead can trick him into thinking that this is a mode that she can just switch on. He's not only asking for a re-enactment of some kind but to be able to have a little respite from sexual decision making.

At the heart of it, he wants her desire for sex to be visceral rather than passive. It makes sense. Their sex life needs a bit of a shake up and some variety and it never hurts to ask. She might want to go there. But if every fibre of her identity is digging its heels in at the very prospect of dominating, it's just one of those things, like desire, that needs to be shelved for a while.

Your need to stay in control needs to choose how control is expressed.

Let them in rather than trying to let go

Just let go is the call cry advice for women who are yet to taste their own version of orgasm. Permission granting for feeling blocked with arousal and orgasm cannot be surmised with these three words. Many have tried. The command of *just let go* isn't permission granting, because it's a command, and the female libido isn't a switchboard with a fat controller perched behind it. So take those three little words and shelve them. If they haven't worked for you before, they probably won't in this moment.

Here's what I propose. Rather than letting go, could you shake it up and make it more about letting someone in? When control is necessary and the idea of letting go and surrendering just isn't going to happen, I see letting in as the sweet spot. Similar to what we covered in the *Permission to trust* chapter, letting someone in is a statement of *I trust myself.*

Taking it deeper, it could sound like: *I can let them in because I trust myself.*

When you drop the idea of letting go you simultaneously drop all kinds of pressure from the equation. The same also goes for the need to have sex to mark a special occasion – this is control's shadow at work and it tries to make sex a must for certain occasions as a way of sealing a deal, or conforming to an unwritten law. You'll be more open to letting them in if you don't feel you have to let go.

You can be in control and be held

An unhealthy relationship with control can mean that you mistake being held and supported for being carried.

There's a big difference between being held and being carried.

Being held is temporary. It's nourishing, affirming and acknowledging. Your partner wants to hold you and soothe you. You are worthy of it. You are worthy of rest.

Being carried requires a degree of dependence. In times of extreme need like grief, sickness, conflict, pregnancy and parenting, someone may offer to carry you and this can create a lot of discomfort. Life will come with punctuation marks of needing to be carried and if we ignore these offerings, we can wind up hardened by burnout.

One of the antidotes to your daily life and having your shit together mode of contraction is to allow yourself to be held.

Because us good girls need instructions sometimes, the following are three ways you can be physically held. I have listed them in a way where each one requires more vulnerability than the last.

1) Lying on your side on the bed, have your back to their chest. This allows you to be held by being spooned. Talking is possible in this position and you can say what you want without being seen. Your eyes can be open or closed and you can harness your nervous systems ability to wind down as you lie down. Start with their hands gently enveloping your body with light pressure and if you would like more pressure, use your own hands and arms to tighten their hold on you.

2) Standing face to face, bring your bodies together and hug. Notice if there are parts of you that aren't touching and as the hold proceeds, bring your pelvis to touch theirs; your belly to touch theirs and your chest to touch theirs. Move closer so that there is no space or air between your bodies. Then, allow your weight to drop into their embrace so that they can hold you in every sense. Have only your toes touching the floor as you have your body held in a tight embrace. Breathe slowly and stay there for more than 30 seconds as this promotes oxytocin release. This bonding neuropeptide will encourage feelings of security, safety and love.

3) Full surrender. Your partner sits on the bed with their back against the bedhead and their legs outstretched. You move into their lap and have one of their arms supporting your back and one of their arms scooped under your knees (as if they are carrying you whilst they walk). Gently increase the

pressure of the hold to a squeeze so that you can be cocooned by them. In this position, you can hear their heartbeat, make eye contact and speak to each other.

If being held physically feels too encroaching right now, could you be held within other means like a conversation? By receiving a gift? Through having someone helping you? Or by simply sitting next to you as you cry. These are all acts of releasing and loosening the reins. Play with these new ways of being in the opportunities outside of sex to build evidence that you can have a degree of control over how you are held.

Trusting ourselves in daily life
increases trust of ourselves in sex.

Trusting our partners in daily life
increases our trust in sex.

The edges need to soften and be made malleable. When you front up to your pain, your fear of vulnerability and reluctance to be feminine, you are being responsive and receptive. You aren't in that hardened state that lets old rules and shutdown be the status quo. That alone takes a lot more effort – effort that could be used putting your control to good use.

ELEVEN

Permission to take your time

ARE YOU IN A RUSH?

I know I am. But I'm trying to change that. Or am I? I often find myself doing everything the same way, which is at a frenetic pace. Always at a frenetic pace.

Even though I don't completely subscribe to the approach: *the way you do one thing is the way you do everything*, it does have some merit when it comes to the pace with which we live our lives and how that plays out in the bedroom.

Just a heads up, if you're living fast and you want to witness change within your sexual responses, it's a slow burn.

And we high-achievers/smart girls/good girls/gotta-be-the-best girls are in constant motion. This whole *change your sex life* thing requires patience that we don't feel we have.

In our fervour of getting shit done, we have confused action for being in motion. We waste time trying to move through our sex problems quickly with band-aid approaches only to look back and think, *if I just took my time and did it thoroughly, maybe I wouldn't still be feeling so frustrated. Maybe by now I would be on the other side and feeling a whole lot better than blocked or anxious.*

Our other problem is that we have confused stillness for stasis or stuck-ness. But life and sex call for stillness at times. Without this medicine, that I so often resist, this book would not be in your hands right now. When I shifted my perception from being stuck in my offerings as a sexologist for the need to be still, something BIG could be birthed inside of me and now thousands of women are able to benefit.

We have applied these self-governed laws to not just life but to sex as well. So, while we're at it, let's expose those other two big laws that suppress our expression…

If I am too much of this then it's a bad thing.
If I am too little of that then it's a bad thing.

This is a tricky one because neither of these outlooks motivates us into changing our intimate lives. Notice how there is next to no incentive to be either of these polarities? When what you want to be in sex becomes an either/or, you end up choosing neither. When you choose; or more aptly, default to neither, you wind up doing nothing.

Instead, can you do a little something and take that little something slowly? There's a secret to slow and it's this…

Take your time and get there faster

The ultimate paradox is that taking your time with sexual exploration will get you to your desired feelings faster. Taking your time will let new opportunities emerge. And I'm not talking marathon sessions. I'm talking 30-40 minutes once a week, including the cuddle time on the end. This part is really necessary for letting everything sink in, especially anything that you've done for the first time or done differently.

An extra-added benefit is that it also allows for all of your precious learnings to integrate. There's something jolting and jarring about jumping out of bed as soon as sex is over so if you have the urge to get clean STAT – resist it.

If you can, lie in some of the tender mess that is pure sex – the smells, the fluids, the warmth. It's a really gentle way to practice softening and softening is what so many women are not giving themselves permission to do. It doesn't have to be a big, bold gesture of being swept up like a victim that needs rescuing. It doesn't have to mean being out of control. It can be as accessible as:

Today I will soften into the afterglow of sex,
where I feel the mess but stay in it anyway.

The way sexual enhancement softens us is a process to savour. My clients cotton on to this pretty quickly when they notice that trying to smash through sessions and learnings quickly just won't give them what they need. Ticking the boxes might satisfy their taskmaster mind but their bodies end up taking charge by slowing down the speed of sessions.

The body prefers to learn slowly and considerately.

I can say this with certainty to women who thrive off the rush but they need to feel the beauty of slow in their own body to believe it.

Take Cam. She wanted to have each of her sessions with me weekly in order to get this learning over and done with. Yet each time we booked a session close together, her body, intuition and busy schedule stepped in to rebook and to give her a little more time and space in-between sessions. Because the body knows that rushing and learning don't get us anywhere fast.

The rush and urge to learn is admirable, just we need to accept that our minds and bodies have a different cadence.

Time wants you to respond with it in mind

Time wants you as an ally but it feels you resist its loyalty. It's patiently waiting for you to engage with it but you keep saying: *when I do ALL of this THEN I'll be engaged with you.* It boils down to the fact that everything in life feels like it needs an urgent and immediate response. Interestingly, there are very few things in life that are an emergency yet we keep treating everything as such. Feeling aligned with time means starting to make decisions about what is urgent and what isn't. When we ignore this act of empowerment, your nervous system is left with no other option than to respond to everything on high alert.

This happened so intensely within me in 2012 that I had to undergo cardiac investigations for the palpitations that kept disrupting my…well, my everything. My body would give me that kick in the guts feeling (or more specifically, a jolt within the adrenals) whenever I thought of something I had to do. Problem was, as a high-achieving sexology student that was working in the stressful terrain of drug dependence and undergoing a radical sexual transformation, I felt like I had something that had to be done *all* the time. Whilst I kept my shit together and achieved everything I wanted to that year, my body paid a price. My heart in particular was showing the greatest strain. The palpitations were the cover story. The real concern was that I was betraying myself, my spirit and my libido from constantly operating in this mode of *I don't have enough time – there is always more I have to do.*

Even as I write this with fervour, I need to remind myself that there is plenty of time.

Putting on my nurse hat and now my mama hat, I have become accustomed to putting off simple necessities like going to the toilet and having something to drink because *there isn't enough time to, something is more pressing.*

I'm finally getting how that connects to our pleasure.

Moving slow means feeling more.

I say this for you and for me. Can we all slow down and come to value stillness a little more for what it has to show us?

That scoffing our favourite foods isn't always as pleasurable as savouring them...

That putting off our need to go to the toilet in an effort to save time only creates more discomfort...

That asking our partners head to rise up from under the covers prematurely doesn't get us to our heightened arousal faster...

Taking your time equals respect

Taking your time is an act of respect for yourself and the other person.

I know that I feel immense respect for other women when they ask if they can take their time so that they can make a fully informed decision. If you need to take your time to respond to someone's request or question – sexual or otherwise – and they move into pressuring you or trying to coerce you into saying the answer that they want to hear then you aren't being respected.

Dig deeper and ask yourself if you value and respect others who take their time but fail to hold this as a value for you. If you rush through to answer someone else or people please in your actions, it begs the question:

Am I responding on autopilot by saying what I think the other person wants to hear?

Respect is conveyed most clearly with our words. Learning to communicate with clarity involves trust. Trust will develop and your intuition will be sharpened when you have multiple experiences of pausing, choosing and speaking out in complete alignment.

When Kylie asked me how to turn off the clock in her mind, I asked her what the clock sounded like.

She shared with me that it sounded like she should hurry up and that she should get sex and her orgasm over and done with.

You may have already noticed that female sexuality does not respond well to a clock or a set of rules. So when the mental clock starts ticking to get you to rush through your pleasure and 'get to the point', it calls for a reminder that:

...it's safe for you to take your time

...you are worthy of taking your time

> *...rushing is not going to get you to a pleasurable end point faster*

And if you get blocked or stuck during sex, know that you will need time to move out of contraction.

You need time to move out of contraction

In your need to move fast, contraction may well be your steady state. When we keep forging ahead through life at full speed, our bodies don't feel safe and start to self-enforce contraction to ground us back down into our primal needs of security and belonging. If the concept of contraction doesn't feel familiar to you right now, it operates under several guises.

Contraction is being curled up on the edge of the bed just wanting to be left alone (whilst simultaneously craving to be held).

Contraction is that lump in your throat that has you feeling like you can't speak, even if you wanted to.

Contraction can also present as the sore, tight neck or pelvis that struggles to feel relief.

Contraction is what has you at a standstill in intercourse. You suddenly realise you are frozen because you doubt your abilities and wonder why you didn't get the run sheet for sex. You ask yourself, *what are the steps I need to take for this to be deemed a success*?

When contraction comes up in the midst of sex, I've found the most effective way to acknowledge it and to move through it is to pause rather than stop.

Permission to pause

Language has the potential to enhance or end your sexual experience all because of the way a thought cascades down into your body. Needless to say, so many of us are stuck in the agonising realm of complete frustration with our limiting thoughts and negative mindsets on a loop. Before you start getting frustrated about feeling frustrated, know that…

Frustration means that you care.

When the feeling of frustration strikes in the midst of sex getting started, it works to put the brakes on pleasure. It catapults our big core fears into reality, namely, worthlessness and powerlessness.

How many times have you needed to stop sex, whether it's at the very beginning of it being propositioned, midway or when penetration or oral sex is already happening?

When you need sex to stop, it's usually because your guard has gone up and your bodily armour has been activated. Let's be clear, this is a necessary response to protect you.

But what if I said you could work your way out of this one in a gentle manner?

What if, when you are safe in the arms of your loved one or safe with yourself, you paused rather than stopped?

This is about giving you another chance to shift gears rather than having your sexual response play out on the same loop. Our bodies and minds are habitual creatures and every time we stop sex at the same or similar point, we inhibit our growth from that place.

Stopping denotes all efforts being abandoned.
It spurs more frustration and self-loathing.

Pausing allows something else to blossom.
It gives respite and a chance to reset.
It births creativity and honours self-worth.

I'm a huge advocate of this approach because I have felt the power of pausing in my own sex life. More often than not, it's been a case of sex being propositioned by Ed and I instantly feel the familiar tug of hearing the *yes* of my desire and the *no* with my arousal or vice versa. All I know is, something isn't lining up for me and when that happens, I crave alignment like it's the only balm that can soothe. Sometimes, I haven't listened to my body from the get go and have gotten flustered, only to take a breath, regroup and say: *sorry, can we try again?* That is the power of the pause in the moment. It creates another opening.

Other times, I let him know that sex isn't going to happen right now. This is still a pause but it's really more like a delay. The usual culprit for holding me back in that moment is the fact that I'm still well in the midst of a high-grade stress response. What that means is that my internal stress levels are too high to be receptive to sex. I could try but the fact of the matter is, I know that I will kind of fuck it up later with some version of sabotage. I'm human like that.

So here's what I do to move through the delay. I talk. I express. I release. I usually cry about something that is causing my self-worth to drown. It could be small or enormous. Doesn't matter. The point is I get it out rather than let it eat away and leech from my precious libido.

And after 20 or 30 minutes I feel better. I've cleared. I feel held by my man just listening. In that moment, I don't need problem solving. I need acknowledgment.

My clients love the concept of pause rather than stop because it gives them choice. Anxiety, shutdown and aversion mean that you stop everything in sex because you have gone into contraction. More specifically, something has happened or a defence has been triggered that has caused you to go into self-protection.

Stopping in sex can be necessary but if it's the default in that it always happens, it means you aren't getting to what's on the other side. It means that connection and the build-up of arousal falls flat because anxiety wins.

When you need to pause, always, always use your slowest and deepest breath as an opportunity to come inward, reset, buy some time and start again from a place where you feel comfortable – it might be receiving a foot rub, hearing your partner hum a song or say something you really need to hear or smelling an essential oil. On that note, using the same oil each time you feel this way can work as a signal that you are safe. I personally like Sandalwood when my root chakra feels unsafe, Lavender when I need calm and Cypress when my throat wants to open.

All of these actions segue to what else is possible and can be used in isolation or as part of a sequence. My experience is that it improves my chances of feeling connection and pleasure, as my actions go to meet them rather than they come to me.

Know that your pause may be long

Permission to take your time means that you may decide at some point or several points in your life to put sex on pause for a long period. The decision to pause from sex for days, weeks, months or even years isn't the same as stopping when it's an informed and aware decision to be celibate or is taking place to honour personal healing. Most notably, this pause from sex altogether is a necessary chapter after heartbreak and separation or for the first few months after giving birth. We need time to heal and as healing as healthy sexual expression has the potential to be, sometimes there isn't a place for it when we're processing something profound, painful, traumatic or unexpected.

Heal in whatever ways you need to and trust that your libido and desire for sex will return in due course. Move through what you need to with grace first.

Should you find yourself questioning if the pause has shape shifted into a stop, take a moment to feel if the empowerment of choosing to pause instead feels like you are being blocked. Feeling stuck, in a funk and as though there is something wanting to crawl out of your body and spirit will be key indicators that you need to come back to sexual expression. Acknowledge that you needed the pause to heal but it's turned into a stop that has begun to limit you.

You can wade back into the waters of giving and receiving and unfurl to sexual permission granting gently again, rather than forcing to be all on for sex and intercourse. Kind and heartfelt touch from your own hands or someone else's are perfect for reawakening your senses and to practice coming back into the realm of the erotic.

When you feel tempted to pace your re-emergence quickly, know that you have permission to take your time.

TWELVE

Permission to sabotage

IT WAS A SERIOUS SESSION but we both ended up cutting through the tension with a hearty laugh. We were looking over what we had discussed the previous session. Amy and I had curated a plan to help her initiate sex that night. It was daring but she had the fire in her belly to do it. She got in the car with a hop and a skip and within seconds, she was talking herself out of it. When her man arrives home that night, instead of greeting him in the negligee like she had discussed in the session, she withheld touch and affection and proceeded to pick a fight with him.

A week later, she was struggling to recall what the fight was about, its reason so meagre. When he gently asked what was wrong and if she wanted to go have drinks at a friend's place that night, she escalated. Although he was simply asking if that was something she wanted to do, she immediately took offense thinking that he didn't want to spend time alone with her (making sex more of a possibility). That night, instead of staying in and exploring how they could grow their sexual relationship, they got drunk with friends and hardly spoke.

Amy had a plan to initiate. She had all the steps covered to take her from feeling nervous about it to feeling confident.

So, what happened?

Amy said the words herself in session: "I sabotaged it".

Yup, she did. We then went over everything. She took a deep breath. I had a little giggle. She joined me. It's not that what Amy was saying wasn't important – because it was. I laughed because we humans are so fickle and so predictable in so many ways. Amy's greatest desire at this point in her life is to be in a sexual relationship with her man.

Her greatest fear at this point in her life is to be in a sexual relationship with her man.

It's a classic tale of greatest desire equals greatest fear.

To give a bit of background, Amy is in a very loving relationship but she avoids sex. Before her current relationship, sex had always been used as a sort of weapon for her, which just doesn't cut it when it comes to being with someone she deeply loves. The phoney veneer that let her darkest feelings go undetected by others doesn't have a place now that she's in the realest relationship she's ever had. Up until this point, she hasn't had to be vulnerable and uninhibited without the aid of alcohol. She felt apprehensive about it all and came to sessions to pinpoint what it is she likes about sex, to let go of the blockages rooted in trauma and to work out how she can be truly open with her man.

The more I learn about being a woman and hearing women's sexual stories, the less sabotage surprises me. It's completely common and eerily normal. In all honesty, we women want to be sexual. So. Badly. More to the point, we want to be sexually free…to just rock up and get sex started or to happily go with the flow of our partner playfully grinding against us with a mutual giggle as we wander off to sleep.

So, why do we do it?

Why we sabotage

We sabotage because we're shit scared of what will happen when the sexual woman emerges. We're daunted by the consequences of her being seen. And often, the last person we want to truly see that sexual woman…is ourselves.

Succumbing to sabotage creates a holding pattern that keeps the sexual woman behind the opaque screen. To see her can be likened to a breakthrough: one that smashes everything we've been taught to be true. I see women, my age, younger and older, feel paralysed by the possibility that every message they've received to conform will be shattered leaving nothing but a wild woman. And shit are we good girls scared of our wild woman. We ask: What is she capable of? How can we play her? Is she totally unpredictable?

It all boils down to the fact that the easiest way to keep seeing and being all that we are ready to see and be is to not change anything. So we sabotage.

You know you are sabotaging when you are purposefully holding yourself back from pleasure and what you desire the most. At the heart of it, you most likely sabotage when you don't feel you're worthy of those things.

I see it as though everything is lined up for you – a golden apple all ready for you to take a bite and you'll walk away not only still hungry for it but self-harming for no good reason. In that moment, it doesn't matter if all of your dreams are laid out before you. If you don't think you deserve or are worthy of what you want, you'll do everything in your power to push them away and maintain the status quo.

Your libido is no different. It's your guide and your muse. Your radar and your compass.

We women want to be so intertwined with our libido yet we repel it.

What would it be like to walk up to the mirror, look yourself in the eye and acknowledge that you are a sexual woman that is worthy of expressing this dauntingly real and incredibly ancient part of yourself?

When sex = sabotage

Sometimes, sabotage plays out a little differently when we've already owned the sexual woman inside. When the sexual woman is already comfortable with sex and pleasure, the style of sabotage isn't about sabotaging sex and connection from the outset. Instead it's a sabotaging of her growth, sense of ownership and empowerment *through* having sex.

I did this in my twenties. The pattern would play on repeat – I would grow in my blossoming identity, hit a new level of independence and immediately get back in touch with my ex to have sex and bring it all back down again to baseline. It was a classic tale of using sex to gain love. Despite it irritating me when I witnessed it in other people's lives, when I did it; it was of course, different. Or so I believed. I told myself countless times that my intention was different, that I wasn't using it for validation or to secure loving feelings. I wanted to fuck without attachment when all I needed was to have sex that was rooted in love.

Let's be honest, I wasn't great at lying to myself and pretending to be something I'm not. When that sabotage pattern ran its course and I collected enough self-worth to stop re-exposing myself to triggering scenarios, it's as if the next chapter of my life was given permission to start.

Sabotage eventually gets painful

Sabotage becomes painful when it doesn't feel like it's protecting us anymore. Instead of buying us some time, it feels like life suckage. Time wastage.

Sabotage becomes painful when you realise that you don't have juice in the tank and honestly...you wouldn't want to be around you either.

Movies and TV shows sometimes glorify sabotage in order to stimulate a response of empathy. But the character who sabotages isn't the underdog here. They're the ones that have stopped fighting their own fight. When did purposefully fucking up become cool and endearing?

Your inner heroine will need to stay on the lookout for sabotage to ensure you don't romanticise it in the hope that she will be rescued and healed by someone else. For certain, sabotage and rescue will be a storyline that will be fallen back on for eons to come but that doesn't mean you have to let it play out in your own life.

If you're looking for inspirational female role models, choose the parts of their persona that you want to express and live them out in your own style.

You can be a heroine and not sabotage.

Accept sabotage will keep happening

Sabotage is an inevitable part of any learning experience. I myself have done it so. Many. Times. It's a natural response we humans undertake when we are being edged into new terrain and the way of permission granting to sabotage means that our self-punishment is a lot lighter when we do stuff up. Which, in our own eyes, we will.

Personally, I sabotage when my self-worth is shaken and I don't know where I stand. That inevitable state of limbo that crops up when we are between two worlds is a trigger that I still fall for. Again and again and again.

It takes a while to not believe your own bullshit.

When that tank within you is running low, it's so easy to default into wanting someone to fill the void of your worth. Although I still want someone to save me in those dark moments – even as my mind screams that it wants validation and my ego is clamouring for a hit of recognition – I deep down know that the only way I can close the worthiness loop is via my own acknowledgment and love. It's a moment to call on my sovereignty.

The sabotage-growth-worthiness triad is inherently self-centred. No external source can keep your worthiness circuit up and firing. The people you choose to have in your life do not exist to confirm you are needed and wanted. Instead, in healthy relationships and dynamics, we choose to be together and to come together again and again as two wholes – somewhat fractured and bruised in varying degrees but whole nonetheless.

Moving out of sabotaging behaviours requires rock solid presence, which is almost like *anywhere you'd rather be territory* for your hyper-alert brain. In the case of Amy, we worked out, at a later point, that maybe we overshot the mark by moving more into actioning what she wanted to happen, rather than stepping back and actioning what she needed to happen.

Needs must come before wants.
You need to be comfortable and confident
with your needs before your wants.

Despite her desire to initiate sex and have it flow with her loving husband, Amy needed to have a sense of mastery over her ability to give and receive affectionate touch first. We made a plan to scale everything back a bit and to wade into the waters of sexual touch, by not doing anything sexual at all. She knew this from the outset but couldn't resist following excitement and its possibilities first. It was more attractive than the basics of intimacy.

Realistically, her whole being needed to feel safe and sabotage free with greeting her husband, being held, kissed, and ultimately being vulnerable, before all of that touch and presence could be amplified into something sexual in nature. She needed that first. If we had proceeded to skip her primal need for affection, she would have not only closed up further but any sex she did successfully have would have been replicating an old pattern of giving herself away whilst proclaiming "I don't give a fuck".

Oh, but she does give a fuck. And you do too.

Healing sabotaging patterns needs your exhaustion

Before you change your sabotaging ways, you need to be sick of sabotaging. You need to be dog-tired of doing the same shit on a loop. Without this, you won't have the fire to change.

If you're in a relationship, your partner also needs to be wearing a little thin from your patterns too, unless they are getting some kind of kickback or benefit from rescuing you in the midst of sabotage. And maybe, just maybe, you are hoping they shine a light on it to give you the impetus to change. If this rings true, try to get yourself out of sabotage for yourself, by yourself, first. It's a far sexier way to give yourself permission.

Be the heroine. Always, always be the heroine in your own sexual story.

In the midst of sabotage, you will retract. Your mind will dredge up the old stories you have about yourself and your physical response will act as "proof". Your thoughts might sound defeated as *what's the point* and *you're just damaged or not enough* come up on repeat. You'll need your own rock solid speech already prepared.

When I feel tempted to sabotage, this is how I validate myself and what's happening:

I remind myself of how what I want is right there for the taking, whether it be an opportunity to up level in my work, the chance to stop acting so hard and to be held by Ed, or being acknowledged by a girlfriend with words of affirmation (my love language) rather than having it bounce right off my armour.

I remember that being sullen, although very cool in the nineties, just doesn't do it for me because I want to live my fullest life, not my smallest one. Interestingly, I sabotage less and less, not only as a reflection of my self-worth improving but through learning how to listen to my yes and no and instilling better boundaries. The clearer and more aligned my life is, the less I sabotage. Plus, as I age, drama just gets so boring.

Sabotage breeds in murkiness.
Worth blooms in clarity.

Along the way, you will sabotage less and your sabotages won't be on that big scale of fuck-up like, ending the relationship with the person you actually wanted, or saying no to the liberating travel plans because you didn't think you were worthy of breaking free from monotony.

Permission to move from these monster-sized sabotages, to the micro sized sabotages, means that we not only have less drama but we can move on a whole lot quicker.

One of my specific sabotage patterns, for a long time, has been celebrating feeling like I'm in my power, and really aligned with life, by drinking alcohol. That feeling of being in alignment quickly detours into misalignment when one glass inevitably turns into four glasses, and that feel-good feeling has been replaced by something that feels disempowered.

This micro sabotage isn't going to ruin my life but it reminds me that it's easy to have my libido, which is my power source, slip away from me by the actions of my own hand. It causes me pain and I need to briefly re-examine why I do it, to then move through the next day with as much grace as possible. Then I can come back to a place where I trust that it's safe to feel worthy.

After a lapse into sabotage, my antidotes sound like:

...I am worthy of pleasure with my partner

...I am moving towards opening up

...I am safe, I am safe, I am safe

...Growth is what I want, even if I feel exposed as it happens

...Feeling powerful is what I want and is nothing to shrink away from

Worthiness needs to be unshakable before we move into deserving and desire territory otherwise we will, yup, sabotage it.

THIRTEEN

Permission to speak up

YOU DON'T COME WITH A WARNING LABEL. (Thank goodness for that.)

You can't walk around with a permanent *sorry* on your head. (And nor should you.)

The woman who attempts to control everything that enters and leaves her mouth may as well be shackled. Starving yourself of your truest expression means that your libido will be starved as well. Re-nourishing your libido means first nourishing your body and voice. Both are vital counterparts to your feeling whole.

In order to *be* in sex, you need active full body movement and throat sounds.

Your capacity to release the sexual heat inside of you is eerily similar to birthing a baby. When you birth a baby, you can't do it without moving your body or making sound. OK, you technically can but both help momentum and progress.

The way you respond to arousal in the bedroom is no different. Arousal needs your participation and the best way to get the blood flowing is with motion. Erotica is rife with the words *undulating* and *cried out* for a reason.

To be clear, the leap from quiet good girl to woman who speaks to her *yes* and *no* could be too wide to be comfortable right now. However, a gradual transition from unspoken to speaking out is a realistic path that will cushion the way. The art of speaking up will ruffle feathers and the feathers that get the most ruffled will probably be yours. These are acts of confidence and, at times, defiance.

A word of warning for those who feel tempted to fall back into old habits of serving. You do not start experimenting with speaking up because it will please others.

You start because it will please you and allow you to live a life that is aligned. Honest. It won't always go smoothly but trying to keep things smooth for everyone else right now is creating some serious bumps (and some not so good ruffles) for you.

Own your outspokenness

I own that, even though I talk to people about really sensitive matters for a living, I still say stupid stuff.

I own that sometimes my outspokenness can become so warped in my head that after seeing my friends, I want to write text messages simply saying *sorry*. The real message I am sending with these unnecessary sorry's are: *sorry for being me.*

Countless occasions of witnessing other women say sorry for the most innocuous of things got me so close to my own habits. The parallel was achingly close. Quitting with the sorry's was a decision I had to make. I couldn't hold my own in sex and be magnetic when I was constantly apologising for my existence. That shit had to stop.

I had no idea that talking about sexuality was going to be my purpose and that my voice would be my most valuable tool. In that process of being guided to this very point, I've been essentially re-programmed to become the woman that speaks about sex – for women who can't speak about sex. I assure you, I wasn't born this way. I needed to learn this craft and perhaps you do too.

Speaking up was not my forte but saying multiple *sorry's* was.

The most important learning for my throat and libido was that no one can speak up for me. As I became more sensitive to the occasions when someone did speak up for me (or over me), I felt the sting of disempowerment, like I'd been robbed of the chance to befriend my empowered and sovereign self.

Silence is entrenched but you can release it

Your silence shows up in multiple ways:

> *...Someone asks you a question about what you 'do' and you freeze.*
>
> *...Someone simply asks what you are going to order off the menu and you wonder what it is they want to hear.*
>
> *...Someone says something controversial about a topic where you have a burning interest and it's like your voice is in lock-down.*
>
> *...Someone starts making jokes about bodies and what happens in the bedroom and there is nooooo way you would chime in.*

Your silence keeps your power quiet.

The women that I have worked with recognise these patterns quickly. They are all too familiar with the discomfort that arises when they are put on the spot in conversation. Without preparation, and the subsequent anxiety that barges in with an abundance of doubt, her throat is closed off and she moves swiftly into nod-and-smile mode.

She tells me how the easiest option has always been to agree with whatever opinion or argument is flying thick and fast at the time. I've heard too many times 'it's just easier if I agree with them…' (insert co-worker, friend, partner, family member here).

By the time women want to address their libido,
they are so tired of not being heard.
We'll be heard when we speak up.

You'll be better understood when someone special is privy to who you are inside. Your preferences, your tastes, your turn-offs, your pleasures and your points of view. Speaking up gives you the chance to be a canvas with texture when you allow your uniqueness space to express.

Sometimes you don't even know your points of view, or likes, until you speak to them. When you let the words roll out…

…how about ziplining next month?

…I really want to enrol in…

…my job is traumatising me…

…can we try this in sex?

You will feel where you stand.

Speaking up continues to teach me that what I say, increases the chances that, what I want, will come to fruition purely because accountability is a big incentive for me to get shit done. Speaking up also helps me to categorise what's a jumble in my head, and these insights are deepened when I can use my hands to explain what I see and where everything lays.

Sure, speaking up is scary but I have come to value motion over stasis and me saying it out loud feeds that value.

Life sometimes forces us to speak up

There have been times where being a blank canvas had appeal for me because I could seamlessly blend in. Other times, life edged me way out of my comfort zone to speak up out of necessity.

One of my greatest struggles around not speaking up, and the incessant need to fit in, has revolved around my tinnitus and hearing loss. Not only is the experience of isolation, that comes with hearing loss, so shrouded in silence but to take this stigma further, I'm both young and in the exceptional position of listening to women's most intimate stories. And when women share the deepest parts of themselves, they are often sobbing through the words which, unknowingly creates a challenge for me to really hear them.

Confessing my struggles rather than concealing them is the essence of speaking up, not just once but, again and again. Despite my desire for *all of this* burden to go away, the reality is, it never will. My hearing impairment demands that I speak up and share my shame over and over because people need to know what my unique needs are. Otherwise, my capacity to connect to others is threatened from the start.

When I attend a talk, I can't just sit up in the back of a room and hope that I catch the gist of what is being said. Nope, I've got to go right down the front or ask the presenter to use a microphone.

When I speak to a circle or a group of women, I can't just nod my head and go along with what I think she is saying. I need to ask her to speak a little louder and clearer to ensure that she's not only heard but also understood.

I've cursed this persistent cause of stress between my ears many times over and cried thousands of tears. I would love to declare *I own it* but I'm not in the comfort of ownership yet. The paranoia and shame of being a fraud still lurk.

So, here's my choice. I can see my hearing impairment as something that corners me or I can choose to see it as an important teacher in doing the work. When I consider this strange conundrum of being the trusted confidante who has trouble hearing, I can only trust that I am carrying this load to not only ensure I practice what I preach but to teach women that are speaking to me to speak up. Loud and clear.

Permission to be called by your name

The most definitive way to start speaking up is through correcting how you are addressed by others. Every day in real life and online, you are probably addressed with names or titles that you internally respond to. Whether you show this response outwardly or not is another matter.

Take a moment. Are you tolerating being called a name or a nickname that isn't your own? Your libido hears every form of acknowledgment and is the clearest barometer of whether the way you are addressed juices you up or whittles you down.

The way you are addressed with titles and terms of affection other than your name comes down to the fact that people love labels and categories.

My nursing career endorsed labels no end. Working in mental health, drug and alcohol, and then later studying sexology, it was all about the labels. They are useful and they make sure people get the right treatment and medications. Important right?

The shadow side to labels is their restrictive and reductive nature. In all sorts of situations and contexts, you may have been addressed or address yourself with labels such as:

A woman with vaginismus
A busy mum
A sufferer of anxiety
The patient
Depressed
Desperate
Smart
Perfectionist
Honey
Gorgeous
Sweetie
Lovely
Babe

How have labels shaped your world? Your life? Your truest feelings about yourself?

It's one thing to be addressed with a label and another to then adopt it as the way to describe yourself. The way you have assigned yourself to a label either in the past or right now has everything to do with your sexuality because being sexual is somewhat incompatible with most of the labels above.

Labels are great at communicating messages succinctly, but suck at describing a person as a whole. And you are whole.

I'll still use labels upfront in select circumstances but, when it comes to how I show up in the world, I am really craving to be *Lauren*. It's my name. It's me. It's whole.

When it comes to describing another woman, I believe that the more challenging it is to label her, the more woman she really is.

Because being a woman needs no other label.

If it didn't feel safe to until this point in time, you have a right to be called and addressed by exactly the name you want. Being able to speak up about what you want to be called is empowering. It's another quiet middle finger in the face of tolerance – which is merely putting up with a behaviour that is not aligned with your personal code, usually in the name of making sure someone else is happy or satisfied.

When someone calls you by a name or title that isn't what you want, you inadvertently end up shrinking ever so slightly. You end up pandering to the tone of that name or title. You end up conforming.

When it keeps happening and you have already corrected someone, it isn't a case of mishearing your name or not catching it the first time. It's a power play.

The motive behind it is to call you what they want to call you, not what you want to be called. It's for their gratification, not a term of endearment. If the nickname, or way you get addressed, has never received your seal of approval and it irks you every time you hear it, it has to stop.

This goes for: *babe, lovely, sweetheart, gorgeous, beautiful, lady, dude* and any shortening of your name that hasn't gotten your yes. You'll know by the fact that they address you and you just feel this big internal eye-roll, or a shuddering, or you simply feel pissed off about it. That is your libido speaking for you when your throat feels closed.

The way we address other people has fads and as I write this, women addressing other women as *lovely* is having its peak moment. This has spurred me to say to women, usually in written correspondence, that I ask that you call me *Lauren.* When I hear *lovely*, it feels so sickly sweet and I can feel a gap widening between her and I. Because I'm driven by connection, this fractures that experience for me because it starts the conversation off on unequal footing.

When a woman makes contact with me and I don't know her, I only call her by the name she addresses herself when she signs off on the correspondence. Assumptions that she is *Kate* but she likes being called *Katie* are dangerous and this actually happened to me a few years ago.

A woman whose Instagram handle had KT in it attended a number of my workshops. I kept calling her *Katie* rather than double-checking that her sign in details were actually *Kate.* After the second workshop, she wrote me an email saying…

Hi Lauren,
I just wanted to let you know that my name is Kate and that I don't like to be called Katie but that I don't mind that you call me Katie…

Did I feel a sense of satisfaction with this confession? No way! I felt worse because it was as if she was trying to be clear whilst letting me off the hook. I saw how we can't do both simultaneously. We can't own our stuff whilst we people please. And I didn't want to be the exception to her being addressing by her chosen name. I guessed that she didn't want me to feel bad but I would rather be corrected than have her feeling misunderstood.

So when I saw her the next time, I made sure I called her Kate. Because that is her name.

And if there's a part of you that is saying to yourself, *but I like it when my friend calls me babe* then keep that going – you don't have to change anything. If you feel held by that name, feel safe within that title and respond positively, then it has your permission to stay. But if you're feeling anything but those feelings of acceptance, that's your signal to let that name go.

The key to start speaking up is two-fold

Starting to speak up asks that you first feel worthy of being heard, and that you are worthy of having presence and being acknowledged – just like in my favourite definition of libido at the beginning of the book.

If the thought of starting to be more vocal in your intimate life already has your throat feeling like it's gently closing up, know that you can gently open it by playing with all of this in your daily life first.

Start with the impersonal situations to warm up to the personal situations. Appreciate that, in the end, both need equal attention.

Impersonal. Have you ever received something that you didn't want or didn't order? Have you ever received subpar service or point blank rude service and didn't speak up? Well, you may have already anticipated what I am about suggest. Daily interactions and exchanges are one of your rich training grounds for getting confident with speaking up.

You are worthy of getting what you asked and what you paid for. It's time for you to stop tolerating. If you tolerate poor service, incorrect orders and a lack of acknowledgment in an everyday situation, then you might well tolerate some undesirable behaviour in the bedroom too.

The first time really speaking up is the hardest. I promise speaking up gets so much easier with repetition. I speak up so much more now that I almost feel like I am constantly doing deals and giving feedback to product and service providers. I feel my heart beat, swallow my fear of rejection and repeat: *don't ask, don't get.*

The next time that food or drink order isn't correct or the item doesn't scan correctly at the supermarket, go against the grain of your silence and speak up about it. Feel the discomfort, make eye contact and gently explain the situation. This action alone could be the difference between you enjoying a situation and you sabotaging it.

Personal. You may never feel ready but you'll know when your story is worthy of being heard. Most importantly, your story needs to be heard by someone that you can trust. Until you verbalise the story that lives inside of you – your love, your losses, your trauma, your womanhood, your dreams, you are held back by the true clarity, ownership and sweet release from what's burdening you.

I encourage you to completely open up to another woman, to find your voice and if you don't have a trusted friend yet (she's coming – you will draw her in as you become more confident) then an expert therapist or coach is the best way to go. When you remove that cloak of fear, shame and not enough from your story, you are positioned to move on and call in what it is you want.

Being held by another woman in confidence is the most effective and nourishing way of bringing this skill into your personal sexual relationships. Another woman's empathy and softness for you will teach you how you can treat yourself safely with empathy and softness. We are all here to teach each other – walking through life as each other's permission granters to open and bloom. And above all, we are teaching each other to feel safe in the truth that you can speak up and still be strong in your femininity. Having supportive women in your life is a necessity.

Speaking up commands clarity

Whenever I approach a conversation or an interaction where I fear retribution, my language can become obscure and vague. Not only do some pretty strong nerves have the reins but I'm also trying to soften the delivery of the blow. The problem is that my original message can get lost in a haze of awkwardness and all that is left unsaid.

Before I share with you the words that speaking up depend upon, it feels timely to remind you that being self-centered isn't the same as being selfish (I personally don't think we can hear that too many times). Self-centeredness is a solid anchor that emits clear boundaries so that energy can be preserved.

Being in a state of ownership and self-centeredness requires specific language. The words that deliver unshakeable clarity are:

Yes. No. I want. I need.
Please. Me. I. Stop.

These words don't have gaps or points of infiltration. They are complete and whole. They don't point the finger and they don't hide behind the well-worn armour. Looking at them, they seem so unassuming – they aren't long or complicated and above all, are really common. But that's what gives them this kind of quiet power. So every day, but so hard to say.

By the time I saw Pam for sessions, she was in her mid-fifties and had been in her marriage for many years. From the first session, she began to realise that she had blocks around making sound and speaking up about what she did and didn't want in the bedroom (and her life beyond). In the fourth session, she told me about how she had made a significant shift, all by noticing that her arousal wasn't building and then saying to her husband: "can you please stop?" Now, before we go on, take a moment to observe how we can read those four words as really harsh in their delivery or, at the other end of the spectrum, really softly…almost like a whisper?

Keeping your words certain and delivering them in a way that matches the situation is the craft of the sexual woman.

Back to Pam. Her greatest fear was that speaking up in this way would, in her words, give her husband *the shits*. What actually happened was he stopped instantly and said: "I really like you saying that". All along, he was yearning for her feedback so he could truly please her in the way that she responded best. Her silence prevented this and, instead of protecting him from possible rejection, kept her orgasmic expression on a lower volume. Her request to stop turned out to be a much-needed pause that allowed them to reset and tune into what was going to work for her.

I love how the simple act of speaking up creates openings for intimacy and warmth that just aren't possible when we exist in the void of entrenched silence.

FOURTEEN

Permission to have trauma

If permission to be sexual on your terms was stolen and taken from you.
I am sorry.

If you were denied the chance to find out about your sexuality for yourself first.
I am sorry.

If you continue to shudder at every touch that feels erotic or sexual even when it's years after that violation.
I am sorry.

BEING DENIED THE OPPORTUNITY to explore your sexuality without interference is a grave human injustice. In my mind, it's the gravest injustice because your sense of safety in your body and your erotic power was attempted to be taken from you. I say *attempted* because I don't believe that anyone can ever take everything from us. Your power is still within you, I promise. Power can be replenished, resourced and re-accessed.

Trauma is everywhere and in everyone

Women have experienced individual and collective trauma at every point in time. More specifically, this is a trauma that every woman has *survived,* despite so many odds.

When I use the word *trauma*, I am referencing both what has happened to us personally and what has been exposed to us. This exposure includes what we've witnessed through art forms like film and online videos, what we've heard through personal stories from our clients, friends and family, what we've read and what the news presents to us. Trauma is a collective melting pot rather than one individual offence.

I also use the word trauma to reference any kind of transgression or boundary crossing that has left you feeling taken from, taken advantage of, violated, shamed or where your consent wasn't honoured.

It could have been verbal, physical, sexual, emotional or all of the above.

It could have happened in a medical context, like a surgical procedure or childbirth, or it could have happened in a public space with a stranger. It also could have happened in private with someone you know really well.

You may have been the survivor or you may have been a witness.

Some of you will struggle to recall the exact details of what happened and some of you will question if you can ever take a breath without this *feeling.*

It's safe for you to use the word trauma when you recall your sexual experiences and abuse.

It's safe for trauma to be a valid reason that stops your arousal in its tracks.

Part of this unravelling of trauma, for me, means that I no longer compartmentalise and categorise it like I once did. I now deeply believe that we are all traumatised in some way.

When you have trauma it's inevitable that there will be pieces of it that will never really settle down and never really fit or slot into a designated space in your body, mind and spirit. Naturally, it will surface in our most vulnerable moments because it craves an outlet that's in the feeling realm. Trauma can be more easily contained when we are in our thinking and achieving brain and that's what makes work and purpose so addictive when we are in pain.

If you are thinking, *but I don't have a history or trauma, I've never been abused...* know that your trauma may not have targeted you personally. Despite what we have come to believe, trauma evades categorisation and isn't selective.

The majority of my own trauma is made up of everyone else's trauma (called *vicarious trauma* in psychological circles). It's comprised of the thousands of stories about trauma that I have been exposed to working in the darkest corners of mental health and drug dependence. These stories especially have stayed with me.

My own personal trauma is also rooted in boundary crossings. Like the guy that dropped his pants in the front of me in the library at 7 years old; the old man that asked me intrusive questions about my "sex life" on the train at 14 years old and the mental health client that told me all he knew about me, leaving me shaken and exposed (and on International Women's Day no less).

When you were violated, that created a ripple effect into the heart of every other woman.

Your betrayal becomes ***our*** *betrayal. We all feel it and we all share it.*

Trauma can show up in the midst of pleasure

Trauma is sneaky and inserts itself without permission because our fear centres are fast responders. As much as our brain values pleasure, the desire to survive usually beats what feels good to the punch.

When Ed and I went on a joy-filled shopping trip at the Museum of Sex in New York City, I never anticipated how triggered I would be by something that was meant to be fun. In the hope of bringing more spice into the bedroom, we purchased restraints for our bed and safely packed them away to use when we returned back to Australia.

We landed back home and there was some bubbly excitement surrounding the first time we were having sex because this time was going to be different. We opened the box and got everything set up quickly. I volunteered first for being tied down, curiosity being the driving force for exploring a new outlet for sexual expression. In my hopeful enthusiasm I thought: *this harness could be our new novelty go-to*!

Yet the moment the last restraint was placed on my wrist, my entire body revealed to me the collective trauma, rape, abuse and violation of every story I have ever heard and walked alongside. Ever.

In a nanosecond, every woman's trauma was activated inside of me and it was all so distant from being fun or playful. I became panicked and started saying "no, no I don't want to". Ed could see the distress on my face, untied all the restraints at a lightening fast pace and I went straight into foetal position on the bed. I couldn't talk. I didn't have the words for: *I know we were just being curious and experimental but I feel like I just felt the rape of every woman that ever existed.* I was in stone-cold freeze response.

I wish I could tell this story differently – to instil this rock solid hope that everything you do to try and bring novelty into your sex life will seamlessly become a part of your next sexual chapter. I wish I could guarantee that this novelty or toy or object will be the piece that was missing all along.

The truth is that your old trauma or collective trauma may emerge when you try something new. This emergence might look like running out of the room, shutting down or checking out. It could transpire as being mute or maybe even pushing through the rest of sex because that's what you've always done.

Trauma wants your acknowledgment

Rather than pressure yourself to acknowledge your trauma in this moment, you can say to yourself: *I may allow permission to happen at some point...not yet.* When you allow this acknowledgement, an old voice in your mind might be tempted to minimise your story or put it next to another persons trauma and say, *but…it isn't as bad as theirs…*

Trauma comes to us to be healed rather than we go to it to heal it.

When you come to a point of readiness to acknowledge your trauma, it's as if the tendrils of traumas receive the red light to stop intruding on every facet of your life.

Speaking directly to your trauma by saying: *I know that you are there* won't make it any worse and it won't give it free reign. What it could do is keep it all in check.

The loop of swallowing it down, only for it to keep appearing at the worst of times, needs to be intercepted. This doesn't mean that there's anything you have to do. You don't have to do shamanic healing or intense psychotherapy to heal unless you are being guided to do this. Perhaps right now, a whole lot of healing can come from saying:

I know you are there trauma
I want you to know that I am safe…
that I have a home within myself.

I acknowledge you and I want you to know
that you do not make up all of me.
Trauma, I am here for you now.

This could provide a way of slowing down how your old trauma bleeds into your current sex life. When your brain and nervous system are in trauma, sometimes the distinction between then and now is blurred and in this haze, you start to approach your own sex life with the feeling of it being traumatic.

Could you separate the past and the present a little?

Can you say there is a distinction between the old violations and your current sex life?

Feel free to take it deeper by noticing the difference between:

I am my trauma and my trauma is a part of me

The trauma is now and the trauma was back then

My trauma will stop any intimacy and I will pause when the trauma arises

When a friend and colleague, Nicole voluntarily contributed to this chapter with her own story of giving herself permission to have trauma, I came to learn how important it is that we decide when we are ready to acknowledge it.

She recounted how she didn't want to admit that she had trauma for a long time. Now in her 40's, her journey was one where she didn't see a place for her trauma in her long-term consensual sex life. She noticed that not giving herself permission to have trauma meant that she couldn't truly get over it. When it became the elephant in the room, there was a pivotal moment. She said to herself: *I think I am traumatised.*

From that point I could get help. I have learnt that trauma needs love. If we don't offer trauma what it needs, it will get louder. It wasn't until 20 years later when I hadn't given it any love or acknowledgment that my nervous system said 'oh – you still don't know. You were traumatized.

I felt in fear. I was alone. Lost.

The biggest trauma is not being able to talk to anyone about it because it becomes toxic and turns into shame.

When you aren't giving yourself permission, you are still in the shame of it. We are treading water and are stuck and can't heal.

When I asked her what acknowledging trauma looks like, Nicole said that she visualises a younger version of herself and comforts her. "I wrap my arms around the trauma inside with the energetics of unconditional love.

No one else can tell us what our trauma needs – whether it be words, energy or touch. We need to intuitively offer it ourselves."

You are doing your best

You are undoubtedly doing your best to reconcile and adapt to the pain of trauma that still feels so raw inside of you.

I have no doubts that if you are with a loving partner that you are trying, and have tried, to meet them halfway in your lovemaking.

I understand that an act of sex that held possibility for

excitement can turn so quickly into a replay of your darkest nightmares.

I feel so deeply how unfair it is that what was meant to be fun and pleasurable in that moment is anything but for you.

Your trauma is a valid reason to pause in sex.
Your trauma cannot be pushed through.

It doesn't matter how many times you need to breakdown over your hurt. I'm sure you keep it together the rest of the time.

You are never unworthy when it comes to feeling safe, feeling loved and experiencing all the forms of intimacy. These human rights should never have been threatened in the first place. As soon as you find a skerrick of strength, reclaim these rights of yours.

Know that you are worthy of being loved and held and worthy of sharing your sexual body without shame or disgust.

I am doing my best

Even before I became a sex therapist, the wound of injustice was a big trigger for me to break down into heaving sobs. As a potent combination of being a helper and a Libran who lives life on a set of scales, I'm driven by correcting injustices.

Thinking of all the children and adolescents that have had their safety violated fuels this deep overwhelming sadness and has me asking: *how did sexual abuse and sexual assault not happen to me when it happened to so many others?*

When the injustices weigh down on me, I feel the collective trauma rise and it sounds like this:

Why should I feel good when so many others have suffered horrific abuse? Why should I keep following pleasure when so many others have had their pleasure dismantled?

Nicole gave it a name – the shame of privilege.

It happens. There are times when my body and fear responses can't separate someone's experiences and memories from my own. That is what makes trauma so powerful and everlasting. It's determined to not let us forget so we can avoid recreating those conditions again.

When the shame of privilege arises, I pause, breathe and follow my sexual pleasure with the spirit of reclaiming it. In these moments, I don't want to feel like trauma has won or has stolen an opportunity for me to release in a healthy way. When trauma does feel all encompassing, I try to stay the course of reclamation.

Interestingly, I don't do it for me so much. I do it for everyone that has ever suffered. I come back to the truth that:

When I don't let trauma derail my pleasure,
I can live as a beacon for those that are
still actively experiencing it.

I can't help women to rise and give them permission if I am drowning in collective pain.

I feel your trauma, I do. Everyday. But I can't let it consume me. I will always acknowledge trauma as a part of our human journey but I won't let it constantly override the love and joy.

I hope you too can say the same.

FIFTEEN

Permission to have boundaries

When you've got a massive heart, it beats and bleeds with such ferocity. It does this so it can keep giving to, and acknowledging, others. This can make you all too wary that your actions, especially those from the heart, will cause a chain reaction in someone else.

One too many times, you have taken the fall for another because it boils down to this truth – you don't want someone else to feel something negative or painful if you can absorb it for them. You would rather feel uncomfortable yourself than have someone else feel uncomfortable. You also don't want them to see you in a certain way – difficult, bossy or unwilling to compromise. So you absorb the shock and swallow it whole.

You become the *yes* woman because there is no line between you and someone else. It's blended and merged. Whilst this notion of being completely fused with your lover is kind of sexy in the early stages, as time progresses, being enmeshed doesn't allow for much eroticism to flow. More to the point, you could find yourself looking in the mirror (or avoiding it altogether) because your identity is an amalgamation of peacekeeping and people pleasing. As beautiful as it is for you to flow and dance between different nurturing and caretaking roles in life, you fantasise about getting some relief…

Boundaries provide us with this relief.

The tendency to default to a *yes* response leaves so many women befuddled when their body suddenly answers with a *no* for them one day. Nothing outward has changed but internally, her body has been keeping the score of subtle traumas and invasions.

The body knows what the head can't make sense of. The body always knows where its *yes* and its *no* reside when it comes to sexual propositions and offerings. For as long as we ignore its cries, we will remain disconnected from it.

Boundaries get less awkward – true story

The word *boundaries* entered my lexicon as soon as I started mental health nursing. Often used in the context of clients acting over-familiar in the hospital setting, "pushing boundaries" stems from a place of wanting to be included, connected, loved and needed.

As you may have already experienced, this boundary pushing can be toxic and exhausting.

Understanding it in the toxic sense is pretty straightforward because it's so off-putting you want to avoid it.

Understanding it in the subtler sense is tricker because it can look like you are just being kind or helpful but your intentions underneath may be somewhat different.

And I would know.

Being a helper means that I am deeply caring but can fall prey to taking action to feel needed. I've worked for as long as I could legally work (which is 14 years old in Australia) and all my jobs have been of service to others. Being of service means that you can sometimes lose sight of those finer boundaries because you just want to help people. Only that, sometimes you're helping people who don't want to help themselves.

Even though I had worked in healthcare from 19 years old, come age 26 my personal boundaries were frankly, all over the shop. Now, my life wasn't in complete disarray but there were more subtle interplays of boundary crossing with mutual benefits. In short, we were both getting something out of it. I was susceptible to being in my good girl that didn't really know what she was doing or where she wasn't growing up even when life was beckoning me to.

It took time for me to reconceptualise boundaries as energy preservation.

Working in mental health and drug dependency was a steep learning curve on the boundary front and it didn't stop when I started as a sexologist. Going the extra mile has often been tempting, particularly when I hold concerns about how my business is perceived. It might be going over time in sessions or giving a client an extra email. At the heart of it all is this desire to help but sometimes this is transpiring as being really, really, readily available (I winced when I wrote those words). Whenever I start to feel like I want to push those boundaries open a bit more in order to be kind to people, or if I'm worried about my sense of worth, I remind myself:

I have given and invested enough in that person.
My time is important and I highly value my time.
I highly value my energy levels.

These are some of the very real things that I say to myself. The more I sit with it all, the more I come down into the truth of my libido.

My libido loves to give and it needs fuel for giving in sex.

I worked out that when I want to help people, I'm not helping them when I enable them.

When I used to get worried that I would be seen as mean, it occurred to me that robbing another woman of a chance to learn something for herself was actually the unkind course of action.

When I do things for other people, or even when I protect them from feeling something painful, I'm enabling them and enabling makes them dependent on me – the opposite of ownership. Enabling can be challenging to spot at first because it can look like protection and safety, but now with a lot more experience in truly helping women, the difference between supporting her and disempowering her is strikingly clear.

Learn your no, find your yes

Establishing boundaries is equally about categorising what gets your yes and what gets your no. In the hunt for what gets your yes, your no can be left trailing behind.

When women say *yes* to sex again and again even when they know it's a no, they can start to shut down. By the time I see women privately, they are still in love with their partners but don't get why they don't want to have sex with them anymore.

Maybe they ignored their body one too many times. Maybe they didn't realise it was a no and they felt like they were already in too deep. So many women fear being the cause of their partner feeling rejection.

But here's the thing. When you learn your no, you will find your yes. Your real yes, that has fuel in the tank to give because you aren't living in martyr mode. That's the mode that asks you to give out of habit and obligation.

And if your partner loves, respects and honours you, then they'll wait to meet the woman who knows the difference between yes because she has to and yes because she wants to.

Maybe…

…it's a no to having your ass slapped but it's a yes to having it gently grabbed

…it's a no to anal sex but it's a yes to external anal play

…it's a no to giving oral sex in the bedroom but it's a yes to giving oral sex in the shower

It begs the question: what if some really carefully planned time out from sex could give you the space you need to work out what you like and what needs to go?

Boundaries call for equity, not compromise

Far too often I have stumbled very quickly into the trap of thinking that something is a compromise in a relationship. Compromise breeds resentment and it's as if I see women take a deep breath, look forlorn and say, "we all need to compromise".

If it works for you, great but if like me, it feels kind of unsexy and dry then you and I both need to keep the focus on that little notion that is *incentive*.

I'm not incentivised to compromise because I don't think it's often needed or necessary. It's just that most people *think* it's needed (and that it's the only way for relationships to work).

Instead, I propose this: *equity*.

I visualise my relationship with Ed as one of equity. Equity is about each person getting what is right for them. NOT everyone gets the same (another trap), or the idea that we need to do things we don't like for each other because that's just the way it is.

Equity gives me incentive because it taps into my core ideal of what is fair for each person.

Within my relationship, when we are in the flow of equity we are nurturing our relationship from a place of giving the other what they need because we want to support them to rise. The fact is, sometimes we have the same needs and sometimes they are worlds apart so a tit-for-tat approach doesn't often tally up.

Equity makes room for our changeable natures and lifestyles, which have become multi-layered with the arrival of our girls. We don't always say yes to each other's requests but, because there is a lot of love in circulation, we are usually deeply happy to say yes to that request with some tweaks. To me, equity feels very different to compromise because it's rooted in and honouring of our individual expression.

Just because you can, doesn't mean you have to

When you start living a life that is self-centred, you also start to realise how much you used to do just because you were capable of it.

Or it felt comfortable for you.

Or it felt known.

Being released of bounds that say: *I can do this so I have to do it,* will have you feeling a new lease on life that you didn't think was possible. Some of this ties in with the *Permission to be choosy* chapter but what you also need to know is that there's so much in your life you don't have to put up with or tolerate. Your boundaries don't want you to tolerate, but we'll get to that later.

I started working with Ruth on the back of a major life upheaval. At 43 years old, she could recall the moment, 16 years before, where her parents had asked for her to help with her brother that has a severe neurological condition. Her whole body dropped, she knew the role that was expected of her and in that moment, gave up the idea of ever having a partner of her own. She saw putting the family first as her fate in life and cast having an intimate relationship and having children out of her mind.

It wasn't until 2016 when she had a breakdown at work that she instigated some major changes within her life. She'd always thought it was her duty to help her family but she needed help. When she asked for support and to be relieved of some of her roles and duties in order to preserve her mental health, her parents were supportive. She instilled boundaries such as only going to help her brother when he calls, rather than always offering to help him. In only 6 months, Ruth took back her life for her. That's a pretty short space of time when put in the context of 43 years.

There was no way that space for her intimate life could be felt when her life was filled with service to others. Her libido was all consumed with people pleasing and some boundary violations that she and her family were enabling. Resetting the boundaries was hard but it was a necessary step to self-preservation so that joy and a relationship could take the place of burnout.

Although Ruth's story isn't directly about what happens in the bedroom, it's a mirror that many women resonate with. Choosing to take action and do things just because you can, and not because you want to, is a common trap for when you love to give.

Giving in this way usually feels sustainable until your nervous system stops you in your tracks and says *no more*. In your efforts to be giving, you may have become complacent with yourself and this can create a sense of disgust for what you have always tolerated.

Less tolerating means less disgust

Stay with me if you can. The word *disgust* may come across as a little strong at first, especially when I'm talking about you being intimate with the person that you love. I know I tend to associate disgust with the vile and despicable. But what I've noticed is that tolerating often comes before disgust – those repulsive feelings about sex that see you balk, screw your nose up or feign gagging.

It usually isn't until a woman is feeling disgust about sex with a long-term partner she loves that she will make contact to work with me. To normalise, when couples ask themselves *what happened to us?* it isn't a one-off event that has her turning away from sex, but a series of events, oftentimes appearing small and innocuous. Although several boundary violations are usually at play, I've noticed that the most common one is her saying *yes* to acts within sex because she has always done so. I think the acknowledgment of always saying *yes* needs to come first so that she can unravel disgust, stop what is triggering off that feeling and re-establish her boundaries. Then she can take control within her sex life.

From my work, I have identified several sexual boundaries that I believe every woman has to have.

The sexual boundaries you have to have

I'm all for kink, kook and the taboo but if the following are occurring in your intimate life and you have never explicitly said that they can happen, then they have to stop immediately. The following are serious violations that take place far too often in modern day bedrooms.

#1 Your partner having sex with you when you are still asleep. This is a complete violation of your body and is probably happening because you can't protest and turn your partner down (so they avoid feeling rejected). You're not a sex doll.

The same goes for your partner taking photos of your body when you are still asleep. These will be likely be used for masturbation/self-pleasure and are uncontrolled documents in that you don't know where they will go. If you haven't said yes to any of these, it's a boundary violation.

#2 Being grabbed and groped, especially on your erogenous zones in non-sexual situations where you have already asked for this to stop. It's irritating, annoying and isn't foreplay that will arouse you. Repetitively responding to groping also makes women feel like nags and then they feel like they're in a parent/child dynamic with their partner, which is very unsexy.

#3 Being leered at/watched intensely when you are naked or changing clothes. You can feel the difference. Being leered at, doesn't feel like you are being admired. On the receiving end, there's a subtle threat that you'll be conquered and devoured. If you haven't said yes to it or actively encouraged it, being leered at probably won't get you psyched for sex. If they are the hunter but you don't want to be hunted, being watched will make you retreat and not want to be naked and in your naturalness. That's a killer for sexual confidence and ownership.

#4 Having intercourse vaginally, orally and/or anally when every fibre in your body is saying you don't want to. It doesn't matter the reason, your body doesn't want to do it and the more you push and force, the further you will get from sexual pleasure and satisfaction. Don't hurt or harm yourself in the name of another person's pleasure. You'll likely become resentful.

#5 Bringing someone else or another couple into your sexual relationship where it is a full *no* from you. I've seen this create so much stress for women when all they want is exclusivity and monogamy in their relationship. If this happens when you've said *no* then the situation puts another block between you and your partner rather than work to bring you closer together. Are there other cracks in the relationship that need to be addressed first? Having other people involved can also be too exposing and winds up diminishing any sexual self-confidence or sense of safety you had. Saying *yes* in the short-term could mean your no has a long-term hold on your sexual expression.

#6 Sexual positions where you feel used or acts that feel completely fake and inauthentic to you. If you don't want your sex life to feel like a porno and it's doing damage to your confidence in sex, it's got to stop. If you and your partner really want to see you be sexually liberated and unencumbered then pretending to be someone you're not isn't the answer.

If one or more of the above is happening without your *yes*, it's a call for boundaries to be established. The risk of not speaking up and standing your own ground is that you will feel increasingly frustrated with your sex life and you might even shutdown altogether. More concerning is that these violations can trigger old trauma or create a new one.

Trust that you will say yes more when your no is truly heard and acknowledged.

Establishing your boundaries isn't mean

When you are so accustomed to being helpful, placating others and being there for anyone and everyone when they need you, it's easy to see establishing boundaries as being mean. When we see boundaries as being mean, it's usually because there is some kind of black and white polarity at play, like always being able to help or support is kind and lovely or nice (*shudder:* those words!) but not being available to help or support is cruel, bitchy or selfish.

Give yourself permission to remove yourself from living on a narrow spectrum of good girl/woman/wife and bad girl/woman/wife. Your capacity to give and nurture, help and support isn't all of you, even when you feel compelled to prioritise these actions maybe not only in life but in your chosen field of work as well.

This is a good time to come back to that definition of libido – *your ability to give and receive pleasure, enjoyment and acknowledgment.* When you've got a big heart that has an even bigger capacity to give, it's vital that you start getting comfortable with receiving and getting choosy about who it is that comes into your orb (and who it is that needs to go). You'll still have plenty to give; in fact, you may give with even greater presence and satisfaction. This protection will give your giving longevity.

You are not being mean when you protect yourself.

That may need time to sink in.

You are not being bitchy, and again it's not that you're not nice or not the cool wife (she is the partner that says *yes* to everything); it really just means that if something doesn't feel right in your body and your values aren't aligned with that action then something needs to change because you risk leaving yourself depleted.

Boundaries are a declaration of your worthiness of what it is you want to feel. It's those feelings that drive your existence and will make you libidinous.

Over-stepping your boundaries creates a learning opportunity

The harsh truth of understanding our proverbial lines in the sand is that we usually step over those lines in order to work out exactly where they are. Really, it's almost as if we need those times in the realm of *this is too much* or *this is not good – I'm really fearful right now* or *I don't feel safe talking to them* in order to come back into our truth.

Not feeling safe is your cue that there's a violation of your boundaries at play.

A BIG cue. Remember that being able to open sexually requires your safety. Safety is number one for women. You will learn so much more when you are safe because you'll be in a state of receptivity. If you do slip and over-step, really feel the weight of that violation and rather than have it pull you down, use it to buoy you back to re-establishing yourself.

I've had moments where I have definitely and definitively over-stepped my own boundaries. I've done the nod and smile routine because I wanted to be a good student of sex and life, so I would take all of what this person/guru/teacher had to give on board and continued to disregard my most trustworthy warning signals flashing. Beeping. Screeching. I did this because I feared that if I mis-stepped then I would be relegated to the not-a-good-student or not-a-good-woman pile. Yes, I learnt from them, I learnt A LOT but I don't believe learning and getting clear on boundaries has to start as a sapling in the soils of fear.

If it took going through burnout, and getting exhausted from being in martyr mode, to start to value your boundaries, know that you aren't alone. Boundaries respond really well to maturing, regardless of your age. Rather than dwelling on how much you swayed and diverted to get to this place of being self-centred, keep the focus on how these lines and parameters are serving your identity now and for your future you.

A confident purpose will clarify your boundaries

It's easier to feel and establish your boundaries when you nurture your identity, purpose, passion and curiosity. Once you source what it is that you are here to give back to this Earth, it becomes apparent what needs your laser focus and most precious energy stores.

The more I feel sure of why I'm of value here, the clearer I am, and the clearer I am, the more satisfied I am. Satisfaction allows me to cap my activities, time and boundaries because there is nothing else I am seeking. When this magic aligns, I am satiated and full.

When you are on the path to sourcing your identity, I believe you are susceptible to having excess libido that spills out into others because you are unsure of how to use it effectively for yourself. It's a case of *I don't know what to do with this so I will pour it here, here and here*. When you don't know what you need, your capacity to give can be leaky and needy. Trust that time will reinforce your libido to be clear and consistent.

Get comfortable with your identity and you get more comfortable in sex because you know who you are and you own it.

If giving yourself permission to have boundaries needs an anchor, I would start with this – the nectar of boundaries is that lines in the sand, fences and parameters are acts of kindness and sovereignty. When you are in a giving haze and need to get clear, break it all down into feeling whether your actions are empowering or enabling. Remember:

You are only being mean if you enable them.
When you walk alongside in kindness and equip them
to walk alone, you are empowering them.

And most importantly, empowering yourself.

SIXTEEN

Permission to not use products

HOW MUCH OF A RELIEF WOULD IT BE to not need pages and pages of words like this and instead just purchase a product that will take care of everything?

I'm talking minimal effort.

When you read the sales pages of sex toys and pleasure objects, it can start to sound a little like that is what will happen. You have a problem and this product is the solution.

Can I ask, have you already tried products to solve your problems?

No matter how much you will them to, or how convincing the marketing, a product probably won't be the answer to your real world sexual problems. Sure, your purchase will work as a permission granter and taboo disruptor but it won't change how you feel. I'm talking on a deep, soul level.

Information has this power that products don't.

Expressing through your voice has this power that products don't.

As of now, try to see products more as supplements and facilitators than direct problem solvers.

Your libido is a minimalist

Your libido does not crave for high stimuli environments and the promise of more with toys, dress ups and aphrodisiacs. It wants to be understood on the barest of levels. Stripped back to its essence instead of decorated.

> *Knowing how to breathe when you feel anxious is a superior tool to a vibrator.*
>
> *Knowing when to move when you feel bored may be all the spice your bedroom needs.*
>
> *Knowing that when one touch irritates you that you have another pressure option, will be more helpful than a faux leather whip.*
>
> *Knowing you are confident to make sound on your exhale will bring your arousal up quicker than a novelty lube.*

When you reach for the product before your true problems and trauma are acknowledged, you could be unknowingly contributing to a deeper divide between your libido and giving it what it needs. Approaching your deepest frustrations and inability to "let go" with titillation can not only flare up the problem but also deter future efforts that are actually more effective.

In all likelihood, when a quick fix doesn't work you become deflated. The *not good enough* mindset kicks in and you turn on yourself.

Instead, turn the anger that not good enough generates and invest it in going inward. Use that fire to stir up what inhabits your deepest recesses. I'm talking about all those stale feelings that are lying dormant like powerlessness, guilt and shame. In general:

Products take you out of your body but further into your problems.

Processes take you into your body and move you through your problems.

The news that your sexuality doesn't require much can give you the biggest sigh of relief or, alternatively, cause your heart to skip a beat. If you were secretly hoping that you could use a product to keep the feeling demons quiet then this may cause you to retreat.

It's only temporary.

Coming to terms with what you have been doing and how differently you are about to approach your sexuality can be jolting before it juices you up. What it looks like in action is:

Less Sexpo, more learning.
Less porn, more real life.
Less toys, more introspection.
Less stuff, more choice.

I never thought that I purchased a lot of sex products or toys, but when I included lingerie that was intended to gratify someone else, it turns out I actually had quite a bit of stuff. Now that I'm clear on what I actually need, this is what my sexually minimalist drawer contains: condoms, lube, oil, a dildo, a candle, a soft piece of fabric to enhance sensation, and a glass of water on top. The rest for me is superfluous.

It all comes back to getting serious about your libido before you have fun with it.

Where meaning well goes sideways

When I started to dabble with selling sexuality products during my sexology studies in 2012, it was unsurprising to me that I had a lot to learn and catch up on.

Who ever heard of a woman selling pleasure objects who had never actually used a pleasure object before?

I quickly caught up to what felt like the rest of the world, read the blurbs and moved into being a self-taught vibrator expert. I got my first vibrator. It felt decadent but I never edged into the terrain of being dependent or addicted. Naturally, the vibrator that I became best at selling at pleasure parties was the one I owned. Marketing and sales were always easier when I connected to what I was sharing with other women because it was real to me.

I had received the permission to use pleasure objects but was my life even missing them in the first place?

The answer is no.

When I was selling them, I had women's best interests in mind but I don't believe that requires the sale of an object as verification. I don't believe your very own declaration of getting to know your sexual self requires a product purchase.

Nowadays, when I read the blurbs for yoni eggs, wands, balls and beads, the promises seem sky high. I always take pause to consider the very real physical and emotional concerns of my clients and there's no way that a product purchase will be the key to unlocking their erotic power. There's way too much to unpack before a simple solution can be inserted. In fact, it can stunt their growth by deterring them from trying other workable options.

False hope is a turn off.

This is permission to not part with money to buy an object that will collect dust in your drawers and remind you that you aren't doing enough for your libido.

Products are fun, they enhance. Problem solve they don't.

As I write this in 2018, the movement for female pleasure objects has begun to blur with the overlap of physiological aids intended to support pelvic floor dysfunction and injuries.

Suddenly, practitioners within the sexuality movement are also experts on the pelvic floor and how to improve its functioning without actually knowing if the woman standing before them (or the woman clicking 'buy now' on the PC) has a problem to begin with.

Don't place pressure on an object to heal you.
Don't place pressure on it to open you up.

Check whether you have a problem to solve

Your anatomy has a basic make up that looks just like millions of other women yet your body will contain subtle secrets that only you can unlock.

By now, you've probably heard a little about your pelvic floor – how it supports your sexual and reproductive organs, the way it relaxes to help you wee (and poo), how it helps to birth a baby and contributes to orgasm! The pubococcygeus (PC) muscle isn't a muscle to be overlooked.

Yet in the name of health, the prevailing message is to keep it all tight and toned and that isn't a message that every woman needs to hear.

Too much tightness is not a good thing.

What so many people give little attention to is the hypertonic (or overly toned) pelvic floor.

We aren't all walking around with loose pelvic floors waiting to be corrected by crystals, balls and wands.

Women experiencing pain with sex have quite the opposite problem. Penetration is a challenge because their pelvic floor is receiving the message to stay in contraction. As the pelvic floor is a major muscle group, this pain and tightness can be alleviated with the expertise of a pelvic floor physiotherapist. And if you are looking to ensure that you cover all bases of how your pain influences your beliefs and vice versa, seeing a sex therapist simultaneously will generate the best outcomes.

I say all this because I fell for the trap of tight = better.

One of the products I endorsed most in my short time as a pleasure object saleswoman was a set of Luna Beads. They are two weighted balls encased in silicone that you insert vaginally to enhance traditional pelvic floor exercises. I used them regularly and even participated in a challenge to wear them daily throughout the month because in my mind, more equals better!

What eventuated from daily use was my once perfectly normal functioning pelvic floor became hypertonic. Intuitively, I stopped using them before I reached the point where tampon insertion or penetration became painful but voiding urine was a new experience. The flow would stop and start and I found myself wriggling on the seat to relax my pelvic floor to allow my bladder to open on cue. As I sat on the toilet at work, I realised the beads were the reason. After that, they got put on hold for a while.

I was under the impression that everyone's pelvic floor needed work.

Then, in early 2015, two months after delivering my first baby vaginally, I couldn't keep the damn Luna Beads in. They just kept falling out.

I hung my head. My wise woman emerged that day to comfort the good girl who just wanted what was best for women but didn't know what was best for each woman as an individual.

Yes, products have the power to promote and restore back to health. Whether they have the potential to heal in the midst of dysfunction, pain and distress is an unknown. No doubt, the real answers lie within the variation of individual experiences.

Feeling like anything isn't optimally working within your pelvis warrants a visit to a pelvic floor physiotherapist who can undertake an examination to confirm any suspicions and provide you with functional movements that can help tend to the root cause. Relief may come with or without the use of physiological aids – at least you'll know what it is *your* body needs.

After my second baby, I've needed a combination of both movement and a pelvic floor aid (in my case, a pessary) to enhance my PC muscle recovery. I'm comforted by the fact that they have been prescribed specifically for my body by an expert. And it was my personal trainer who gave me the permission to go and see a pelvic floor physiotherapist. That's the power of one conversation, one mention – a woman can receive the wisdom and healing she needs.

Know the problem before you try to solve it.
There may not be a problem to solve.

When you know your sexuality needs some subtraction

The tendency to add more to an otherwise already over stimulated sex life can wreak havoc on a woman's libido.

When Alex came to me the intention was to address her barriers to desiring her partner. As she went through the list of what videos she had seen, the e-courses she had done, the toy she had bought and the forums she had participated in, I began to question why she needed me. The answer didn't take long to surface.

Adding all the stimuli was a tactic to amplify a perfectly good libido from the ground into the stratosphere. Her partner wanted more and this was effectively closing her up more. The message Alex received was that her libido was *insufficient* and her body didn't respond well to this and so stopped cooperating sexually. Disgust started to reign her sex life because her attraction to him couldn't flourish in an environment of being coaxed and pressured.

What Alex was going through was a kind of sexual burnout. She needed less, not more.

When she saw what was going on and how it was disempowering her, she created some firm boundaries and temporarily separated. Upon reuniting, her request to have her consent honoured rather than being frequently pressured into sex was upheld.

The result was a better quality relationship and higher levels of intimacy. She didn't need any more sex tips. What Alex needed was acceptance, space, boundaries and communication skills. She needed respect and to know deep in her bones that she was loved as a sexual equal, not a sexual object.

Products + Pressure = Shutdown

When you plan the big and not so big romantic events in your life, it's inevitable that the possibility of sex will come up. When you are keen to spice things up with your partner, and they with you, outfits and sex toys are a common bedfellow.

Yet if anxiety is dominating your sex life, this third bedfellow could spell the start of an unravelling. If your body starts to interpret all this extra input as pressure to perform, then negative anticipation and shutdown can sabotage any and all romance from even happening.

I've heard it countless times from women – planning sex for special occasions with the presence of products is a sure fire way to retreat and let contraction win.

As Anna's 1st wedding anniversary approached, she was in such a state of anticipation that she was numb. Feeling numb was a very old response to protecting herself when she felt exposed. There was no one else telling her what she needed to be, or had to do, when it came to her sexuality but somehow, she was putting immense pressure on herself to pack lingerie. Soon, her real feelings about it all started spilling out and her real desires came forward. "I just want to wear my big cotton undies, socks and a comfy t-shirt, not chaffing lingerie that sticks into me. It's so not sexy putting all of this on and for what?"

The rest of the session played out as:

I give myself permission to not wear lingerie.

I give myself permission to be comfortable.

I give myself permission to not have stuff.

I give myself permission to not have to have sex on my anniversary night…

We were bringing true permission into the light by stripping back rather than adding to. Anna's feeling that she needed to have all the things wasn't getting her psyched for sex to celebrate but suffocating any possibility for intimacy.

All any woman needs when it comes to sex is her own, big green, blazing light and her ability to be present with her beautiful body.

Your libido is a minimalist.

FINAL WORDS

I FEEL BEYOND FORTUNATE to have been chosen to write this book. Writing *Permission* has gifted me the possibility of truly living in alignment with everything that I've written here. Permission is a topic you can't fake or stumble your way through, it asks to be lived and breathed.

Throughout the process of writing, I asked myself over and over if what I was conveying was completely aligned with how I was living my own life.

Was I being sovereign?

Was I in ownership?

Was I in alignment?

Was I truly giving myself permission to be serious and in control?

...To be sexual and have boundaries?

...To be choosy and feel safe?

If I lapsed, it would be brief.

If I lapsed from being my own permission granter then it

happened because I am woman – unrestrained, cyclical, intuitive and changeable in nature.

Some of the subtle and not so subtle changes that I made throughout the writing of this book include reducing my tendency to apologise, knowing when to slow down and read more books, getting really specific about asking for what I want, connecting with more women by getting out there, forgoing alcohol when I knew it would make me feel powerless, owning the feminine parts of me I have tried so hard to suppress all these years, and finally resigning from a type of work that didn't align with my soul and had my nervous system screaming: *no*.

And the point of all this permission granting?

It's allowed me to be in my own state of personal health and when I am healthy, I am free. Liberated.

And in your own pursuit for liberation you'll need to continue to give yourself permission well after the pages of this book are closed.

That's OK. We're all in this permission granting thing together and for the long haul.

My deepest hope is that the words in these pages have created a solid foundation for you to give your libido the green light to open and unfurl.

Over time, you may come to notice that you need even more subtle permission granting as new situations present themselves. Please be compassionate with yourself. See each and every one as a reminder of your pledge to live as your own permission granter. Each small challenge and test is an uncovering that gets you closer to the real you.

When the temptation to seek out the all clear from someone else arises, remember that this is one of your golden opportunities to ask yourself first: can I give myself permission?

Permission to dream

Permission to create

Permission to release

Permission to let in

Permission to explore

Permission to go against the grain

Permission to act out of character

Permission to crack open

Permission to put my libido first

Permission to be a sexual woman

Now, there's a little secret I need to let you in on before we finish. Other people will notice you blossoming into your own permission granter. In choosing liberation over shutdown, you will become radiant.

When you give your libido permission to shine in every way, others will probably want what you have. This is the time to enforce your boundaries and to only give where it feels generous for you. People find it hard to resist taking when they so badly want a piece of what someone else has. You may have to call in the words:

I give myself permission to give
only where it feels good

As you move with the notions that resonate for you and live as your own permission granter, you will undoubtedly become more attuned to the instances where other women are blocking their own growth and liberation by not giving themselves permission.

Could I ask that you give her a gift in that moment?

When the temptation arises to give her permission as an invested party, could you bounce it back to her?

THE POWER OF:
What is it you need to hear?
What is it you need to give yourself the green light to do or feel?

...changes the dialogue and allows her to step up.

Advice giving and wisdom sharing are integral to our connections as women.

I just can't help but wonder what would it be like if every woman sitting across from us had one brief moment of being witnessed in the power of being her own permission granter?

That one action could potentially create ripples that move into our hearts, bedrooms and lives, making us all...

Less guarded, more trusting

Less victim, more responsive

Less dependent, more in ownership

Less passive, more active

I see it as a world of women harnessing our own individual strengths to move through and move on from suppression and chronic resistance to our own power. Simply because...

Permission is empowering
Permission is trusting
Permission is opening

Permission is the first step to liberation.

REFERENCES + MUST READS

Daedone, N. (2011). *Slow sex: The art and craft of the female orgasm.* Grand Central Life & Style.

Komisaruk, B., Beyer-Flores, C., & Whipple, B. (2006). *The science of orgasm.* Johns Hopkins University Press.

Lister, L. (2016). *Love your lady landscape.* Hay House.

Nagoski, E. (2015). *Come as you are* . Simon & Schuster Paperbacks.

Perel, E. (2007). *Mating in captivity: Sex, lies and domestic bliss.* Hodder & Stoughton.

Thomashauer, R. (2016). *Pussy: A reclamation* . Hay House.

Vitti, A. (2013). *WomanCode* . Hay House.

Winston, S. (2010). *Women's anatomy of arousal: Secret maps to buried treasure.* Mango Garden.

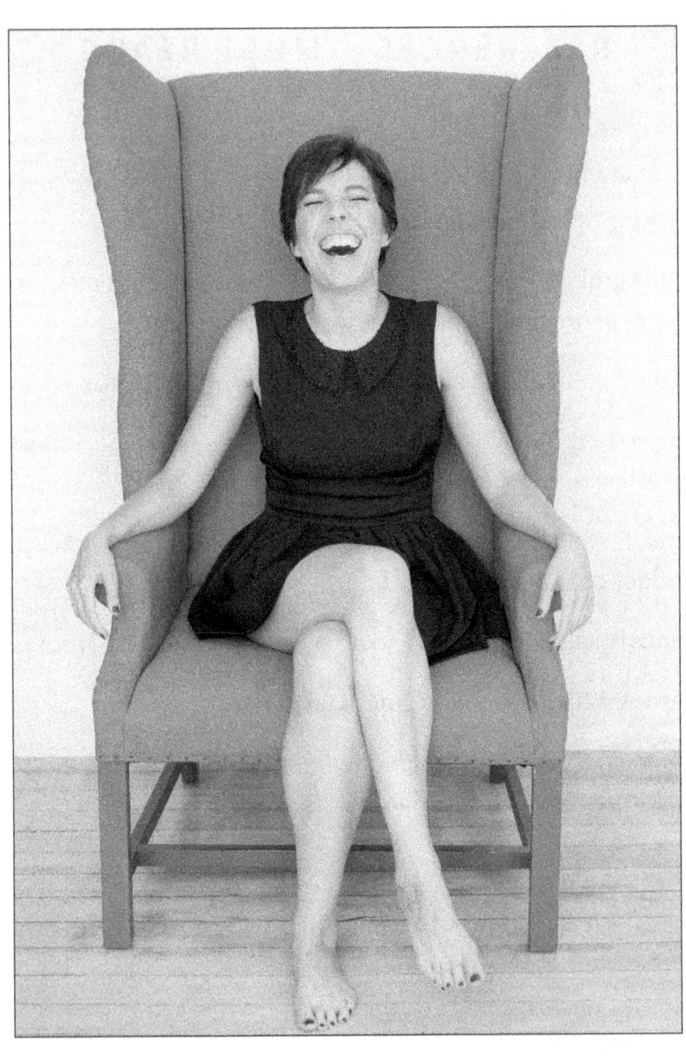

ABOUT THE AUTHOR

Lauren is a qualified sexologist, devoted mama, balanced Libran and lounge room dancer extraordinaire who assists her many satisfied clients to drop the anxiety and reinvigorate their sexual power in their intimate lives. Through her one-on-one sessions, writing and events, she helps women to release their physical and psychological blocks so that they can liberate their libidos for intimacy, sex and life.

For more about Lauren and to access free content, videos and journal prompts for each chapter, go straight to the **Permission Book Club** at www.laurenwhite.com.au/permission-bookclub.

Instagram @laurenwhiteau
Facebook @laurenwhiteau

Share your learnings, experiences and AHA moments with *Permission* by using the hashtag #permissionbookclub so I can acknowledge and honour you.
www.laurenwhite.com.au

www.ingramcontent.com/pod-product-compliance
Lightning Source LLC
Chambersburg PA
CBHW032124020426
42334CB00016B/1059

* 9 7 8 0 6 4 8 3 9 9 2 4 7 *